To Jean Robinson

and in memory of my

Hugh and Charlotte M

TOWARDS THE EMANCIPATION OF PATIENTS

Patients' experiences and the patient movement

Charlotte Williamson

This edition published in Great Britain in 2010 by

The Policy Press
University of Bristol
Fourth Floor
Beacon House
Queen's Road
Bristol BS8 1QU
UK

Tel +44 (0)117 331 4054
Fax +44 (0)117 331 4093
e-mail tpp-info@bristol.ac.uk
www.policypress.co.uk

North American office:
The Policy Press
c/o International Specialized Books Services (ISBS)
920 NE 58th Avenue, Suite 300
Portland, OR 97213-3786, USA
Tel +1 503 287 3093
Fax +1 503 280 8832
e-mail info@isbs.com

© The Policy Press 2010

British Library Cataloguing in Publication Data
A catalogue record for this book is available from the British Library.

Library of Congress Cataloging-in-Publication Data
A catalog record for this book has been requested.

ISBN 978 1 84742 744 1 paperback
ISBN 978 1 84742 745 8 hardcover

Cover design by The Policy Press.
Front cover: image kindly supplied by Jay Simmons.
Printed and bound in Great Britain by Hobbs, Southampton.

Contents

List of figures and tables

Figures

Tables

Glossary and abbreviations

AIMS	Association for Improvements in the Maternity Services
APRIL	Adverse Psychiatric Reactions Information Link
challenging interests	interests held by corporate rationalisers
clinician	health professional in clinical or therapeutic relationship with individual patients
CHC	community health council
conservative	generally accepting the status quo as it affects a particular social group
consultant	most senior hospital specialist
corporate rationalisers	a category of people who promote cost-effective care for populations of patients, not for individual patients; includes managers, health economists and others (see Chapter Two)
doctor	usually a clinician, but can include public health doctors
dominant	exerting the most power or influence
dominant interests	interests held by clinicians, but corporate rationalisers' challenging interests are becoming increasingly dominant
IDDT	Insulin Dependent Diabetic Trust
interest	a stake in something that the holder values
lay people	people with no qualifications in medicine or professions allied to medicine, for example, nursing or physiotherapy
NAWCH	National Association for the Welfare of Children in Hospital
oppression	a sense of being at an unalterable disadvantage, routinely discriminated against, coerced
'ordinary' patient	patient who is not a patient activist

patient	person in a clinical relationship with a health professional and receiving healthcare (may or may not be ill or suffering from some disease or disorder)
patients	sometimes means the plural of patient, sometimes used as a collective term for all those on the patient side of healthcare (patients, past and future patients, patient groups, patient activists/advocates/ representatives) for whom there is no satisfactory collective term
patient activist	patient or former patient trying to improve healthcare for other patients and so politically engaged with the health service; usually means a radical patient activist, unless the term conservative patient activist is used
patient advocate/ representative	patient activist speaking for the interests of other patients and intending to convey a particular view or set of views to influence other people's opinions or actions (see Chapter Seven)
patient group	patients with a shared interest in a specific aspect of healthcare who have formed a group
patient representative	*see* patient advocate
PLG	patient liaison group
primary care trusts	the NHS organisations that purchase healthcare for given populations
public	people who may be patients at some time in their lives but are not patients in the specialty or situation being considered; people in general; citizens
radical	prone to challenge the status quo as it affects a particular social group
RAGE	Radiotherapy Action Group Exposure
repressed	checked in advance, prevented from speaking or acting

repressed interests   interests held by patients and often hard to identify, articulate or promote

user   person making use of health services from time to time while not being in a continuous clinical relationship with members of its staff; an ambiguous term little used in this book but sometimes preferred to 'patient' by people with chronic or recurrent illnesses or disorders

voice   give words to, often used to mean repressed interest holders speaking about their interests or views

Preface

The bits of fur from under the legs of many foxes will in the end make a robe.

(Chinese proverb, quoted in Charles Elton, 1942, Preface)

Sixty years ago, there were no patient groups and few people who could speak for the interests of patients when they conflicted with those of healthcare professionals or managers. Now patient groups are so common that we recognise them as a new social movement. I have been privileged to be a member of various patient groups and of various statutory health service bodies and professional and managerial bodies associated with the health service. So I have both taken part in the early days of this new social movement and observed reactions to it. It has been exciting; it has also been puzzling. The intense commitment and determination of many patient activists, patients working to improve healthcare for other patients, have been plain. Patient activists' proposals about how healthcare could be improved have met with unpredictable reactions from healthcare professionals and managers. Some have accepted activists' proposals willingly, others have opposed the exact same proposals implacably. At the same time, lay people (lay people who are not patient activists) charged with monitoring standards of care or with the governance of health service bodies have often seemed indifferent to the quality of the services. Uncertainties about who can speak for or represent the interests of which particular patients or category of patients are common. These confusions are a sign of conflicts, some well recognised, others scarcely put into words.

For a long time, I have tried to understand what lies beneath these passions and confusions. From experience and observation, from collecting little tufts of fur from many foxes of different shades of russet, I have come to think that the patient movement is an emancipation movement. Some of its members have acted with persevering opposition to some aspects of the status quo, just as members of recognised emancipation movements have acted. Their actions have evoked the same sorts of mixed reactions of admiration and acceptance or scorn and resistance that have met activists in recognised emancipation movements. Other similarities between the patient movement and recognised emancipation movements can be seen, once they are looked for. In this book, I explain what I mean by emancipation and offer evidence that the patient movement is an emancipation movement. Seeing the patient movement like this could give us a new and constructive way of looking at certain aspects of healthcare and at how to improve its quality, as both patients and health professionals would define it.

A few preliminary points.

First, this book is chiefly about the radical part of the patient movement, not its whole, though the two are closely connected, as Chapter Three relates. So I have concentrated on patient groups and individual patient activists whom I know to be strongly radical, that is, who consistently engage in opposing the status quo of current healthcare practices and standards, if they think that they harm patients' interests.

Second, I have largely excluded patients with physical disabilities or with mental disabilities or illnesses from the book. They already have well-recognised liberation (emancipation) movements. Patients here are those in clinical relationships who are not necessarily ill at all (immunisation, screening, childbirth, for example); patients with acute illnesses or disorders; and patients with chronic or recurrent diseases. Patients like these are not usually thought of as in need of liberation; but some of them have formed radical patient groups.

Third, I have not stressed the supposed or proven clinical benefits of offering patients information, choice, shared decision-making and other aspects of care that patient activists define as good, described in Chapters Six and Seven. From their earliest days, some patient groups have drawn on evidence that the policies, practices and standards they wish to see in place can have good therapeutic effects. This sort of evidence is being sought increasingly and being found by researchers independent of the patient movement. It is important. But it is not fundamental to the case for the sorts of standards that radical patient activists want. The absence of a provable therapeutic benefit for any specific standard of treatment or care proposed by patient activists does not itself undermine the merit of the standard. So for the purposes of this book, I have usually omitted therapeutic benefits.

Fourth, books depend partly on their publishers and I pay tribute here to Jo Morton at The Policy Press for the grace and the efficiency with which she has worked on this book.

Finally, I want to acknowledge with gratitude the help I have had from patient activists and from health professionals. Some I have worked with in local or national working groups and committees. Some I have talked with down the years. Others have read and checked what I have written about them or their patient group. In the last two years I have visited and talked with many activist and professional colleagues and former colleagues to ask them questions for this book; and they have been most generously hospitable. I am immensely grateful for their insights, enthusiasm and friendship. I specially want to thank: Priscilla Alderson, Peg Belson, Alison Blenkinsopp, Mitzi Blennerhassett, Mary Bruce, Beverly Collett, Nadine Edwards, Heather Goodare, Elisabeth Hartley, David Hatch, Nancy Hill, Jenny Hirst, Christine Hogg, Donald Irvine, Gerry Jackson, Ann Johnson, Peter Kennedy, Millie Kieve, Paquita McMichael, Jan Millington, Catti Moss, Jean Robinson, Ann Seymour, Sheila Shinman, Andrew Smith, Madeleine Wang, Michael Wang, Helen Williams, Patricia Wilkie and Joan Woodward. My niece, Charlotte Mitchell, gave me good advice and my husband, Mark Williamson, gave me invaluable help by reading every chapter, some several times.

Charlotte Williamson, December 2009

ONE

Introduction

To become a patient was to relinquish a part of oneself, to be received into a system, which, however benign, subtly robbed one of initiative, almost of will.

(P.D. James, detective novelist, 2008, p 11)

Preliminary thoughts

In this book, I argue that the patient movement is an emancipation movement. This idea can seem shocking at first. It seems to deny that health professionals commonly act with expertise and skill, with kindness and care, and from a wish to do what is ethically right and morally good. The word emancipation calls to mind harsh and unwelcome ideas like oppression and injustice. Oppression and injustice can seem irrelevant to healthcare as many patients daily experience it. Moreover, in the UK, we rely on the health services not only to care for us when we need their care, but also to symbolise our concern for other patients. The idea of emancipation seems contrary to these personal and social goods.

The definition of emancipation in the *Shorter Oxford English Dictionary* can help us reconcile these apparent contradictions. The word emancipation comes from the Latin: *e*, from; *manus*, a hand; and *capere*, to capture (Little et al, 1936). In Roman times, masters could keep their slaves in fetters or set them free. Nowadays, emancipation is used metaphorically to mean setting people free from the coercive control or constraint of more powerful or dominant other people or social groups, from subjection to them, from their 'intellectual, moral or spiritual fetters' (Little et al, 1936). Patients are people in clinical relationships with clinicians, receiving healthcare from them. Patients in western countries are not slaves. But patients in 20th- and 21st-century healthcare are in many ways less powerful than doctors and other autonomous health professionals and, politically speaking, subordinate to them. Patients are sometimes subject to various obvious or subtle, open or hidden, coercions and restrictions to their opportunities and abilities to act autonomously in accordance with their views of their interests and of their responsibilities to themselves and to other people. It is those coercions and limitations to patients' autonomy that emancipation can be thought of as being from. Emancipation does not mean rejecting what is good about a dominant social group, those of its ideas and actions that free people from hardship, want, fear, disease or pain. It means altering the relationship between dominant and subordinate social groups, lessening the opportunities for the one to harm the interests of the other. It means adding to the equality, the freedom and the responsibility in the world. In that, it benefits the social group that is more powerful as well as the group that is less powerful. We can see these processes and their results in recognised emancipation movements like the women's movement and the black civil rights movement, even though progress towards equality is slow and halting.

Emancipation movements are not revolutions. Their members have no wish to destroy the people from whose unequal power they seek release. Most feminists do not wish men to have to suffer as women have suffered, nor wish to silence men nor annihilate their masculinity (Heilbrun, 1990). Patient activists, patients trying to improve healthcare for other patients, do not want healthcare professionals to lose their skills, their expertise and their sense of self-worth. Patient activists respect professionals' wish to do good. They wish patients to share professionals' power, making healthcare better for both patients and professionals (Williamson, 1999a).

Emancipation movements are also not consumer movements. In the 1980s, the idea of patients as healthcare consumers seemed to promise higher status and greater power for patients. Consumers or customers want sellers of goods and services to offer them access, information, choice, safety, representation and redress: the principles of commercial consumerism (Potter, 1988). Surveys show that patients want these things from the health service (Chapter Ten). But patients also want the health service to offer them support, equity, shared decision making and respect (Chapters Six, Seven and Ten). These principles are irrelevant or antithetical to commercial consumerism. Some aspects of healthcare can be sold and bought, and all have costs in resources and in human effort. But the purposes of healthcare are different from those of commerce. Healthcare tries to protect or restore people's ability to fulfil the purposes of their lives, in spite of the illnesses, disabilities and injuries that none of us choose but that most of us experience. Healthcare should be guided by moral and ethical values and principles, not by commercial ones like competition or financial incentive (Tudor Hart, 1998). Emancipation movements, in appealing to equality and justice, appeal to ethical values.

In saying that the patient movement is an emancipation movement, I face the difficulty that only some, probably only a few, of its members see it as such. Members work mostly from intuition, that is, from unarticulated knowledge, and from conviction. The patient movement lacks an ideology, a set of ideas to guide its members' actions and to explain them to other social groups, an ideology that reflects 'hope and virtue', in the words of President Obama (Obama, 2009). The movement is still young, immature and fragmented (Chapter Three). It has scarcely developed the theoretical underpinnings that would support any ideology. Yet it is possible to regard the patient movement as an unrecognised emancipation movement: and I do. But that prompts the question, if the patient movement is an unrecognised emancipation movement, what is the evidence that it is an emancipation movement at all? I think that there are four lines of evidence, two direct and two circumstantial.

Four lines of evidence

1. *Direct evidence: the actions of patients themselves, the issues that they identify and the directions in which they seek to secure change*

   From the time in the late 1950s and early 1960s, when patients or patients' relatives began to form patient groups, these groups have been diverse. Some have been formed for mutual support, some to press for more resources or more research or more professional and public understanding for their particular sorts of patients. Others, a minority, have sought to free patients from coercive policies, practices and standards in healthcare. This is apparent in the way these groups have singled out some particular policies, practices and standards rather than others to criticise, challenge or oppose.

   ◊◊ They criticised hospitals for preventing parents from visiting their children in hospital freely, not for inadequate plumbing in the wards or the clashing colours of curtains (as members of hospital governance bodies sometimes did). They challenged the policy of keeping healthy newborn babies in nurseries away from their mothers, in spite of their mothers' wishes, not midwives' practice of keeping an eye on the babies. They opposed the practice of entering patients into clinical trials without their knowledge and consent, not the value of well-designed clinical trials. ◊◊

At the time, these patient groups saw their challenges to policies, practices and standards of care as attempts to raise the standards of healthcare (Chapter Six). But looking back, we can see that the effects of the changes that the groups wanted to make were to reduce health professionals' and managers' coercive control over patients or their relatives. The effects were to increase patients' and relatives' freedom to act as they thought right (Chapter Four). Self-determination and freedom from coercion constitute autonomy (Jensen and Mooney, 1990). (There is a fuller definition of autonomy for patients, patient autonomy, in Chapter Six.) When people act from intuition, from unarticulated knowledge and values, the point at which effects and intentions can be separated from each other can be obscure. So it was here. But there came a time when what these patient groups were seeking could be seen to be autonomy for patients (Williamson, 1992).

The pursuit of autonomy for a particular social group is one mark of an emancipation movement. Emancipation movements work to increase their social groups' autonomy, both that of the social group's individual members and that of the social group itself (Heilbrun, 1964; Williamson, 1992; Epstein, 1996). To do that, emancipation movements have to go against, oppose, some of the accustomed beliefs and ways things are done in society at a given time, some aspects of the status quo: they have to be radical (Chapter Three). Patient groups who seek to change policies, practices and standards in ways that decrease coercion and increase patients' freedom to act, can be called radical patient activist groups. Their members, together with independent radical patient activists, can be called radical patient activists.

This line of evidence was the first to strike me and is perhaps the strongest of the four. The rest of the book gives many examples of what radical patient activists do to try to secure respect and support for patients' autonomy, by proposing specific policies, practices and standards of care to replace coercive ones. Radical patient activists unpick part of the tapestry woven by more powerful, dominant social groups and try to weave a new pattern into it.

2. Direct evidence: patients' laments that they are not treated as people

Again and again, year after year, since patient groups began to note it in the early 1960s, patients have lamented that they were not always treated as 'a person', as 'a real person', 'as a person with a mind', 'as a fellow human being' (Jolley, 1988; Bates, 2001). Exactly what each patient meant by these words is hard to say. But it was to do with their sense that their moral agency, their will and their capacity to take right action, their autonomy, was not recognised or respected. They felt that they were regarded as inferior beings, as non-people.

At first sight, this is odd. Medicine and nursing, and the other autonomous or semi-autonomous professions, dedicate themselves to the welfare of patients. But powerful dominant social groups attribute traits and characteristics to subordinate groups that justify or rationalise their domination of them (Fuchs Epstein, 1988). Thus men have seen women as having inferior intellects to men's and as lacking the ability to reason in abstract ways (Fuchs Epstein, 1988).

◊◊ Many men in Britain in the 19th century did not see women as able to contribute anything serious to men's lives. Mr Arabin, an otherwise admirable clergyman in Trollope's *Barchester Towers*, published in 1857, thought that 'women generally were little more to him than children. He talked to them without putting out all his powers, and listened to them without any idea that what he should hear from them could either actuate his conduct or influence his opinion' (Trollope, 1995, pp 163–4). ◊◊

When the medical profession became effective in treating disease in the early 20th century, the profession became powerful (Gray, 2002). It developed a collective view of itself and of patients (Parsons, 1951). Patients, by contrast, had only their personal circle of relatives and friends, and their own doctors; they were not in communication with other patients like themselves; they could not form a 'solidity collectivity' or group, as the influential sociologist, Talcott Parsons, pointed out (Parsons, 1951, p 477). Parsons held that, ideally, doctors knew best and that patients should relinquish their usual responsibilities and cooperate with their doctors and follow their instructions (Parsons, 1951). Relinquishing responsibility means relinquishing moral agency. Always uncritically obeying doctors' instructions means suspending autonomy of thought and action. How far patients in the early part of the 20th century in fact behaved in these ways can be questioned. Very ill patients may still fit Parsons' ideal (Chapter Two). But by the 1960s, some patients felt responsible for themselves, their families and their communities. We know this from the early radical patient groups, as well as from ordinary observation and from later research into patients' views (Alderson et al, 1994). By the 1960s also, some patients challenged, disobeyed or tried to change professional and institutional instructions. If they had not, there would have been no radical patient groups, no radical patient activism.

Exactly what denigratory traits and characteristics healthcare professionals attribute to patients today, and how far they do so consciously, is also hard to judge. Certainly, some patients feel that being patients puts them at risk of being treated as if they were not worthwhile persons. They devise stratagems to fend off this risk.

◊◊ When she had a baby, this patient took an avant garde novel into hospital and laid it open on her bed, ready for the consultant obstetrician's ward round. She had no wish to be treated differently from or better than the other mothers in the ward; but she wanted to ensure that the consultant regarded her as an intelligent, responsible person (Diana Smith, personal communication, 1996). ◊◊

Other stratagems include joking with the doctors; taking the initiative in saying "good morning, Dr [name]"; mentioning that their spouse is a consultant at another hospital or a member of the same hospital's staff – if he or she is (personal communications from these patients, 2006; 2008). Conversely, some patients whose status or knowledge might seem threatening to doctors, for example, being another doctor or a lay member of the General Medical Council (the body regulating the medical profession), conceal their status (personal communications from these patients, 2008; 2009).

Such deliberate decisions about how to present oneself indicate patients' unease with their status as patients. If patients feel that their status as a worthwhile person, a person with moral agency and responsibility, has been affronted too far, they may take action. One kind of action is to write an account denouncing the care, the institution or the medical and nursing staff (Chapter Three).

Another kind of action is to start or join a patient group (Chapter Four). Forming a group can be the beginning of what comes to develop into an emancipation movement, when eventually some members of those groups begin to wish to claim equality of intellect, of feeling, of moral status and of power with members of dominant groups. We can see this pattern in today's radical patient groups' actions, even though they seldom explain their actions in ideological or philosophical terms. (A few do, Chapter Three).

Once radical groups of any kind (of women, black people, patients, homosexuals, people with disabilities) are formed, they begin to identify new issues, new causes for disquiet, in some of the assumptions, customs, practices and standards that have hitherto be taken for granted by themselves as well as by everyone else. So points 1 and 2, the two lines of direct evidence, are interdependent.

3. *Circumstantial evidence: historical*

The patient movement has grown from small, scattered patient groups, each with its own objectives. This is true both of the movement as a whole and of its radical component, radical patient groups that question, challenge or oppose certain aspects of the status quo.

◊◊ To stop hospitals preventing parents from visiting their children in hospital; to reduce unnecessary surgery on women; to stop general practitioners arbitrarily striking patients off the lists of patients for whom they care; to stop radiologists using vastly different doses of radiation for the same clinical condition, were just a few of radical groups' diverse objectives. ◊◊

These objectives are also examples of how radical patient groups' first objectives are often specific and limited. A few people get together to try to change some specific aspect of the way things are. It is not until later, sometimes many years later, that more abstract, general and ambitious objectives begin to emerge. Then groups can compare their ideas and find that they have themes or objectives in common (Chapter Six).

This, too, is the way recognised emancipation movements began. Their early members probably seldom foresaw that, in times to come, their actions would be seen as part of the start of a much larger whole. We all sometimes act without understanding the potential significance of our actions: the actions create the meaning. Perhaps, indeed, the people who take the first actions in pursuit of their immediate objectives cannot see further ahead in the beginning. It may be the first few steps themselves that 'open [the door] to vistas which would have seemed too glaring before', as the social psychologist Hans Toch, an early writer on social movements, said (Toch, 1965, p 238).

◊◊ After the abolition of slavery in the US in 1865, ex-slaves needed to find paid work. Providing education and vocational training for black people in the Southern States, a cause supported by some white people in the Northern States, were the first steps

—

that led ultimately to the black civil rights movement (Franklin, 1947; Toch, 1965). ◊◊

◊◊ The women's movement that seemed to emerge from nowhere in the mid 19th century in the US and the UK had had precursors in the late 18th century. Mary Wollstonecraft, for example, in *A Vindication of the Rights of Women* (1792), had described women as oppressed and argued for equality between them and men, using the phrase 'emancipation from the galling yoke of sovereign men' (Wollstonecraft, 1975, p 33). Other women had started to ask for education and for the right to work (Miles, 1988; Freedman, 2001). Women had begun to learn to separate their interests from those of men (Miles, 1988). ◊◊

Though I have cited these examples to show that small beginnings can lead to great ends, they also suggest two other points. One is the importance of education to members of subordinate social groups. The other is the ability to examine critically dominant groups' claims to act in the interests of subordinate groups, to distinguish between interests that are compatible with each other and those that conflict. An ability to separate analytically the interests of dominant groups from those of subordinate groups is an early, radical step in freeing the subordinate group from the dominant group's intellectual, moral and political fetters (Chapter Two).

As we have seen, the first steps that lead ultimately to an emancipation movement can be difficult to interpret at the time. Experience, observation and analysis need to accumulate before emancipation movements can be seen as such. Furthermore, interpreting the radical part of the patient movement as an emancipation movement may be hindered by people's unwillingness to contemplate the harsh and unwelcome ideas noted in the first paragraph of this chapter. Or it may be inhibited by people's unconscious emotional or ideological alignment with health professionals, and hence their difficulties in separating patients' interests from those of health professionals (Chapters Two and Eight). This means that it is essential to be clear about exactly what emancipation in healthcare means. Otherwise, patients' and professionals' feelings of shocked defensiveness will prevent them from understanding it.

4. Circumstantial evidence: theories from social science

The first three lines of evidence come from observation and interpretation; they are empirical. The fourth line is theoretical. Political and social scientists have depicted the distribution of power among the main groups of people who hold interests in healthcare – clinicians, managers and patients – in various ways. All social scientists agree that patients are the weakest group in western healthcare, subordinate to more powerful groups. But in particular, one sociologist, Robert R. Alford, has come up with a depiction, a theoretical framework, that I think explains well how the subordination of patients, their subjection to dominant social groups, came about and is sustained (Alford, 1975). As patients gradually become less subordinate to dominant social groups, the emancipation of patients can be seen as a logical extension of that theory. Other social scientists and political scientists, creating theories about how society works, have also put forward ideas, generalisations and insights that can help to illuminate and partly explain some of the actions, relationships and puzzles that we can observe in healthcare. The next chapter discusses some theories and insights that I have found useful in coming to the conclusion that the patient movement is an emancipation movement. In Chapter Two, I also define some of the terms that I shall use in the book. Readers who prefer to get on with the story, so to speak, can skip that chapter, perhaps coming back to it later.

These four lines of evidence can be related to each other in arguing that the patient movement is an emancipation movement, and I draw on aspects of them throughout the book.

The plan of the book

The rest of the book develops my hypothesis that the patient movement is an emancipation movement, mainly by describing various aspects of it and comparing them with parallel aspects in recognised emancipation movements. Some, perhaps all, of the parallels could apply separately to other social movements. It is the combination of them is significant.

So far, I have used the dictionary definition of emancipation. In Chapter Three, I give a definition of emancipation and of the patient movement as an emancipation movement in healthcare. Liberation, a word that people sometimes use instead of emancipation, means the same thing: set free from bondage or oppression (Brown, 1993). I think the first term suits healthcare better because it seems more precise, more likely to remind people that emancipation is from some aspects of healthcare, not from all of them.

Various aspects of healthcare could be drawn on to support the emancipation hypothesis, but here I look mainly at standards of treatment and care. Standards are descriptions of specific aspects or actions in healthcare, practices to which prescriptive values are attached. The values may be quantitative, 'Visiting times are from 2.30pm to 4pm daily'. Or they may be qualitative, 'You must respond honestly to any questions the patient asks'. Or they may be a combination (Chapter Six). Standards can be drawn from any field of knowledge, thought or experience, from scientific research to intuition (Williamson, 2000a). Healthcare works through standards, though they may be explicit or implicit; formally written down or informally passed from person to person; cover a multitude of actions or leave some actions uncovered; be regarded by those who carry them out as important or as trivial, as necessary or as unnecessary; be explained to patients or hidden from them. Standards are healthcare in action. What is done or not done and how it is done gives patients their most direct and personal experiences of healthcare.

Both the actions and the values attached to them are usually chosen by healthcare professionals, but with increasing input now from health service managers (corporate rationalisers, Chapter Two). Whoever determines standards controls a large part of healthcare. When radical patient activists believe that a specific standard, or the absence of a standard, could threaten patients' interests in some way, they try to get it changed, if they can. They criticise it or they suggest some other standard. They may criticise the action or seek to change the value attached to it, or both. Extending visiting hours in a hospital from 2.30–4pm to 2.30–6pm changes the value. Keeping newborn babies by their mothers' beds instead of in a hospital nursery changes the action or practice. In their efforts to improve healthcare, activists try to change various sorts of standards. When they try to change standards in directions that would increase patients' opportunities and abilities to act autonomously, we can see emancipation at work.

The rest of the book goes like this: Chapter Three, The patient movement, is about the beginnings of the movement in the early patient groups who started in the 1960s to try to change standards of care. It draws a distinction between radical and conservative patient groups, a distinction crucial to the proposition that the patient movement is an emancipation movement. Chapter Four, Radicalisation, is about the experiences of healthcare that can radicalise patients. Chapter

Five, Radical activists' new knowledge, discusses the knowledge that radical patient groups create and use to argue for change. Chapter Six, Values, principles and standards, examines the values and principles that give radical patient activists their sense of direction in their work. Chapter Seven, The ten principles, looks at ten of those principles, taking examples from recent or current conflicts between patient activists and health professionals or managers. Chapter Eight, Conflict and schism, offers some evidence from research that suggests that the radical–conservative distinction, first postulated for patient groups in the US, can be discerned empirically in UK groups and underlies some of the conflicts within the UK patient movement now. Chapter Nine, Allies and antagonists, brings in radical health professionals, professionals who, like the men who supported the women's movement and the citizens who opposed the slave trade and slavery, act against the interests of the dominant social groups to which they themselves belong. The support of such traitors or heroes is probably essential for emancipation movements. Chapter Ten, Achievements and failures, assesses to what extent radical patient groups and activists have succeeded in their emancipatory task. Chapter Eleven, What next?, suggests that it is time to flag up the patient movement as an emancipation movement. That could clarify some of the confusion that surrounds patients and the patient movement. It could help professionals think about how they, not only patients, could benefit from the emancipation of patients. It could give theoretical underpinnings to policy makers', professionals', managers' and patient activists' endeavours to raise the standards and the quality of care in the health service.

The idea of emancipation challenges many of our comfortable assumptions. But it may be a necessary challenge if healthcare is to do justice to those who give it and those who receive it.

TWO

Setting the theoretical scene

Modern medicine combines liberating potentialities with oppressive realities.

(Howard Waitzkin, physician and sociologist, 2000, p 37)

Introduction

Emancipation movements seek to throw off the fetters of coercion and constraint that are liable to be imposed by dominant social groups on subordinate social groups (Chapter One). In political language, they seek to free groups of people from oppression, from the unjust use of its power by a dominant group against a weaker one (Mansbridge, 2001a). This chapter shows that patients can be subject to domination and oppression, then discusses Alford's political theory and some other political concepts that can help us to understand domination and oppression, and related concepts like repression, as they can affect patients.

Emancipation movements

Emancipation movements are concerned with differences in power between dominant and subordinate social groups and with the unjust use of the greater power (Mansbridge, 2001a). *Power* is the ability to bring about significant effects, specifically by furthering the person's or social group's own interests or by affecting the interests of others, whether positively for good or negatively for harm (Lukes, 2005). The feminist literary scholar Carolyn Heilbrun said that emancipation movements question the arrangements between strong and weak groups and work to change them (Heilbrun, 1990). The changes that emancipation movements bring about give more power to the weaker group than it had before and, at the same time, challenge both the forms and legitimacies of power in society (Heilbrun, 1990). Steven Lukes, the sociologist who wrote a classic analysis of power, *Power: A radical view*, said that sharing power to protect each group's interests rather than letting unshared power harm those of the weakest group must be the long-term objective of any society (Lukes, 2005). *Equality of power*, of shared power, must be emancipation movements' long-term objective.

Justice is more difficult to define. The political theorist Iris Marion Young defined injustice as the institutionalised conditions under which people cannot develop and exercise their capabilities as individual people, communicating and cooperating with other people (Young, 1990). (*Institutionalised* means the patterns of thought, feeling and behaviour that are largely taken for granted within a particular social institution.) The two primary forms of disabling constraints that give rise to injustice, Young said, are domination and oppression (Young, 1990). Domination easily becomes oppression. To secure justice, institutionalised domination and oppression must be lessened and ultimately abolished.

We readily see certain social groups or categories of people as institutionally oppressed and pervasively disadvantaged. They include women, members of ethnic minorities, homosexuals, people with mental or physical disabilities (Young, 1990; Thomas, 2007). But we are slower to see that patients, too, can be subject to institutionalised domination and can experience oppression. Perhaps this slowness is because we are all patients from time to time, whatever our race, gender or social status. Whether we consult our general practitioner about a sore knee or are rushed to hospital with suspected appendicitis, being a patient is a normal part of everyone's life in western societies. Moreover, when patients are adults (as distinct from children or people with certain disabilities), their ability to exercise their capabilities and to communicate with other people are usually already well developed. So injustice for patients must be defined by looking, not at the development of capabilities, but at their exercise. Then, *injustice for patients* can be defined as *the institutionalised conditions under which they are prevented from exercising their capabilities and responsibilities as individuals and as members of society, to the extent that they are able to and wish to.*

Disease or suspected disease bring with them anxiety and fear. Illness can be painful and debilitating. Treatments can be taxing, death anguishing. Respect and support for the patient's, and their relatives', capabilities, for their autonomy, not threats to it, would seem to be what patients should expect in a humane and therapeutic health service. Domination and oppression are contrary to that.

◊◊ To demonstrate that patients or their relatives can be subject to injustice, inequality, domination and oppression, we can look at 'scandals' that took place at Alder Hey Hospital in Liverpool and the Royal Infirmary in Bristol in the 1980s and 1990s (Royal

Liverpool Children's Inquiry, 2001; Bristol Royal Infirmary Inquiry, 2001). The 'scandals' were that doctors, in seeking parents' consent for post-mortems on babies and children, did not tell the parents that some of their child's organs might be removed and kept, never to be returned, before the body was given back for cremation or burial. When parents discovered that this had happened, they felt that their trust in the doctors and the hospitals had been betrayed (Royal Liverpool Children's Inquiry, 2001). ◊◊

The practice of not telling lay people and patients that organs might be retained after post-mortems had been going on, unknown to patients and the public, since before the creation of the NHS in 1948, and continued thereafter (Richardson, 2001). Taken in conjunction with other revelations that, at Bristol, cardiac surgeons had continued to operate on babies and young children, in spite of knowing that their mortality rates were higher than those for the same surgery carried out in other hospitals, the exposure of the post-mortem practices had significant consequences. Procedures for post-mortems were changed and the 'scandals' contributed to the reform of the system for regulating medical practice (Irvine, 2003; Underwood, 2009).

I shall use political terms (in italics) to bring out particular aspects of the organ-retention 'scandal'. The doctors (pathologists, clinicians, medical researchers and medical teachers) had been able to arrange ways of doing things to suit themselves, and to keep them secret, because they were members of a *dominant* social group. Other people, like pathology laboratory technicians and undertakers, knew that children's bodies were given back without all their organs to their parents, but kept silent (Richardson, 2001). Dominant ways of doing things are dominant because other people accept them (Alford, 1975). The parents' *interests* in their children's bodies and in their own moral agency were *repressed* because they had no means of knowing what would happen or of saying what they thought about it, or wanted to happen to their children's organs: the parents' autonomy was not respected. Their lack of opportunity to defend their own interests treated the parents *unjustly*. They were treated *coercively* because, when they decided to consent to a post-mortem on their child, they made a decision they might not have made, had they known about the possible retention of the child's organs. The parents' moral agency was further affronted because they were denied the opportunity of acting altruistically, if they wished, by giving their child's organs to research or teaching, to benefit other children. When the parents discovered what had happened, some were unassuageably angry, for they were experiencing *oppression*.

Looking at this politically does not mean that doctors had thought about this practice in this way. They believed that their secrecy spared relatives distress, though they were aware, too, that relatives who knew the details of post-mortems might refuse consent (Bristol Royal Infirmary Inquiry, 2000). Doctors' motives seemed to them morally good, saving parents distress, and ethically right, securing organs for teaching and research.

The dominance, oppression and coercion evident at Alder Hey and Bristol were a consequence of doctors' power and patients' powerlessness. Most political scientists agree that in the mid 20th century doctors were dominant and patients subordinate in healthcare (Alford, 1975; Harrison et al, 1990; Salter, 1999; Waitzkin, 2000). The success of modern medicine in treating disease had both greatly improved doctors' status and power and had enabled them to say that their status and power were necessary for treating disease successfully (Gray, 2002). Though political scientists agree with these points, they hold different theories about the details of the distribution of power in healthcare. The theory that I think most closely matches and illuminates what we can see in our western healthcare today was put forward by the American sociologist, Robert R. Alford, in his book *Health care politics: Ideological and interest group barriers to reform*, published in 1975 (Alford, 1975). In outlining it, I add some points from recent commentators.

Alford's theory

Alford studied the failures of attempts to reform healthcare in New York City in the late 1960s and early 1970s (Alford, 1975). Alford used the concept of social structures, a controversial concept among social scientists and perhaps a puzzling one for other people. *Social structures* are the social, political, legal, economic, cultural beliefs and institutions of societies and the taken-for-granted relationships, especially power relationships, between them, that hold societies together, constraining people yet giving them the means of acting with apparent freedom (Sharrock and Watson, 1995). 'Social structure' is a metaphor from plant and animal anatomical structures and means 'the mutual relation of the constituent parts or elements of a whole as determining its peculiar nature or character' (Little et al, 1936). Society is imagined as the whole body; but the parts of a biological body do not necessarily work smoothly with each other, and nor do those of a social body. Both can be changed, biological structures by evolution, social structures by social action. Social action can both reflect and bring about changes in people's moral and ethical sensibilities, changes that can lead to emancipation movements.

Alford divided people who hold interests in healthcare into three main categories of interest holders. *Interests* are difficult to define but roughly mean a stake in something that is important to the interest holder because of the benefit or harm it can do to that person or to the social group to which he or she belongs (Lukes, 2005). *Values*, the worth of something to a person or group (Little et al, 1936), are closely linked to people's view of their own or their social group's interests: if someone values something, he or she holds an interest in it. Alford's three categories of interest holders were:

1. **Clinicians**: health professionals in clinical practice, especially doctors, having or seeking clinical autonomy and concerned with individual patients. Their interests were *dominant*.

2. **Corporate rationalisers**: a diverse set of people including officials in government health departments, executive managers in health services and health service institutions; public health doctors (as distinct from clinicians), health economists, deans of medical schools and many other academics and commentators on healthcare. They were concerned with populations of patients and with the cost-effective use of resources, not with individual patients. Their interests were *challenging*, because corporate rationalisers challenged clinicians' power.

3. **Patients and the community**: their interests were *repressed*, kept from being articulated and promoted, by the other two sets of interest holders.

The interests of any two or of all three of these categories of interest holders could coincide or conflict with each other. When they coincided, who had the most power did not matter. When they conflicted, it did matter: the most powerful group's interests prevailed. All interest holders could support some of the interests of other groups of interest holders, even if they conflicted with the interests of their own social group (Alford, 1975). Repressed interest holders tend to support dominant interests (Chapter Three), but some dominant interest holders support repressed interests (Chapter Nine). Such shifts enable social change, including the emancipation of repressed interest holders, to take place without revolution.

These categories are worth looking at in detail, with examples of how interests and interest holders affect patients.

Dominant interests and clinicians

Dominance means having the chief authority, the most influence, ruling (Little et al, 1936). Clinical professionals' interests were dominant because they served and were served by wider social structures: society's and professionals' interests coincided (Alford, 1975; North, 1995). As dominant interest holders, clinicians had authority to say what healthcare should be; to diagnose disease and prescribe treatment; to define some errors in treatment and care as allowable; to secure compliance with their own policies; to veto those of other interest holders; and to disregard others' preferences (Alford, 1975; McCaughrin, 1994; Salter, 2004).

The medical profession claimed to know what patients' interests were and to act altruistically in those interests. This was apparently unquestioningly accepted by patients and society. Medicine was paternalistic, that is, its policies and practices 'restricted the freedom and responsibilities of those dependent on it, patients and relatives, in their supposed best interests' (Royal Liverpool Children's Inquiry Report, 2001, p 369). As an *ideology*, a statement of beliefs to guide members' actions and explain them to the outside world, the profession's claim that it acted in patients' interests served doctors' dominant interests well, as long as patients and the public accepted doctors' definitions of their, patients', interests. Once patients, the public and social scientists began to question those, to look at them critically, the ideology began to fail. It survives to some extent to this day, in our hope, when we are patients, that doctors will act in our interests, if for any reason we cannot express them ourselves. The ideology survives also in patients' wish to trust their doctors and in doctors' wish to be trusted by their patients (Irvine, 2003). But even *trust* has political aspects, because the more someone is trusted, the more freedom he or she has to act without question or hindrance from other people.

Nowadays, we expect patients to define their own interests. 'It is for the patient, not the doctor, to determine what is in the patient's own best interests', stated the General Medical Council (the profession's regulatory body) in 1998 (General Medical Council, 1998, p 9). This is a significant, and an emancipatory, change from half a century ago. Patients may find, however, that defining their own interests is not always straightforward. They may lack the information they need to judge what their interests are in a particular situation or predicament, unless all the relevant information is offered to them. It is not always offered (Chapter Seven).

Clinicians as dominant interest holders have considerable power to act in accordance with their patients' interests, as their patients would define them. They often do so act, even when clinician and patient do not explicitly discuss the patient's interests or wishes.

◊◊ General practitioners (GPs) can disregard local or national guidelines for referring patients to a specialist, by referring the patient earlier than the guidelines say. For suspected bladder cancer, for example, the GP can refer the patient after blood has been found twice in the patient's urine instead of after three times. Most patients would probably want to be referred earlier rather than later. But GPs who refer many patients who turn out to have nothing wrong with them risk censure from managers and sometimes from hospital specialists. ◊◊

Or clinicians as dominant interest holders can use their power to the harm of patients' interests. Lukes, writing about dominant interest holders using their power to deny the interests of weaker interest holders, said that power as domination 'is the ability to constrain the choices of others, coercing them or securing their compliance, by impeding them from living as their nature and judgement dictate' (Lukes, 2005, p 85). The phrase 'as their nature and judgement dictate', applied to patients, echoes the ideas of personhood and autonomy I touched on in Chapter One and earlier in this chapter, because patients whose autonomy is respected and supported are free to make the choices they think or feel would be best for them.

◊◊ In the early 1980s, it became evident that some clinicians were writing 'do not resuscitate orders' in some patients' notes, without the patients' knowledge or consent (Doyal and Wisher, 1993). This breach of patients' trust (and, as some would see it, affront to ordinary social values) led professional organisations to issue guidance on the subject (British Medical Association et al, 2001). The guidance stated that the patient's wishes should be ascertained (British Medical Association et al, 2001). Now, however, terminal sedation, giving sedative drugs to patients so that they remain unconscious, getting weaker and weaker, until they die, perhaps a few days later, raises the same issues. Terminal sedation is sometimes carried out without the patient's or relatives' knowledge or consent (Harrison, 2008). The rebirth of old issues in new practices is a mark of dominant interest holders' power to choose how they shall act, without regard to what anyone else may think. ◊◊

Medical dominance holds for every level of healthcare. Clinicians can successfully oppose the government's agent, the Department of Health, in negotiations (Salter, 2004). Clinicians in hospitals can refuse the requests of managers.

> ◊◊ A manager in the Accident and Emergency (A&E) Department of Stafford Hospital asked a doctor to stop treating a seriously ill patient so that he could treat several less seriously ill patients, in order to reach a target that no patient should remain in A&E for more than four hours (Healthcare Commission, 2009). The doctor refused. But he was worried that a more junior doctor might have felt compelled to comply (Healthcare Commission, 2009). ◊◊

Individual clinicians can, to a certain extent, choose how they give care to individual patients, through the policies, practices and standards to which they work. Whether one thinks doctors' dominant power protects patients or harms them depends partly on the circumstances. Refusing to stop treating the seriously ill patient protected that patient. But in the first example, some people might regard terminal sedation carried out without the patient's knowledge and consent as an illegitimate use of dominant power, not excusable as an error.

Challenging interests and corporate rationalisers

Corporate rationalisers are diverse (Alford, 1975). Identifying what sorts of people were likely to be corporate rationalisers was one of Alford's most acute insights. The categories are worth noting because academic commentators and researchers seldom declare their political alignments and so may seem 'objective'.

Corporate rationalism is roughly synonymous with managerialism and with bureaucracy. *Challenging* means accusing, calling to account, questioning, summoning to a contest (Little et al, 1936). Corporate rationalisers challenge clinicians over their use of resources, because corporate rationalisers seek the rational use of resources for defined populations of patients, not for individual patients (Alford, 1975). Corporate rationalisers value and have interests in planning, coordination, cost-effectiveness, regulation and audit (Alford, 1975; Freidson, 2001). In pursuing these interests and values, they seek control over the professional and clinical work of clinicians (Harrison and Pollitt, 1994; Freidson, 2001).

In the 1940s and 1950s, corporate rationalisers lacked power compared with clinicians. But when social, economic and political structures began to change in wider society, the distribution of power in healthcare began to change (Alford, 1975). By the mid-1960s, health service executive managers and officials were prominent in the US and were challenging clinicians' dominance (Alford, 1975). They became significant in the UK after 1984, with the government's introduction of General Management (Winyard, 2003).

Corporate rationalisers sometimes support patients' interests against those of clinicians, though not necessarily for the same reasons as patient activists would support them.

◊◊ When the control of decisions about when parents could visit their children in hospital was transferred from clinicians to administrative staff (managers) at the Hospital for Sick Children in Toronto, the administrators de-restricted the visiting (Callery and Luker, 1996). Managers probably acted to improve the hospital's public relations, rather than from psychological understanding of young children's needs (Young, 1992). ◊◊

Here, managers freed parents and child patients from oppressive coercion.

Or corporate rationalisers support clinicians' interests against patients' interests (Chapter Ten). Or they pursue their own interests to the harm of patients' interests.

◊◊ The Department of Health, corporate rationalisers at national level, introduced a *Quality and outcomes framework* in 2004 (Department of Health, 2003). It enabled general practitioners to earn extra money for carrying out some procedures but not for others. Whether it has improved clinical practice is controversial. However, the Department does not oblige doctors to disclose to their patients which procedures earn the doctor money and which do not. So patients may be unaware that their doctor's actions ("I'll just take your blood pressure") and advice are not necessarily based solely on the doctor's judgement of the patient's clinical need (Wilkie, 2008; Williamson, 2008b). This is covert coercion. ◊◊

Power relationships continue to shift in the US and UK, with corporate rationalisers gaining power relative to clinicians, so that corporate rationalism is, in some ways, now ascendant over professionalism (Harrison and McDonald, 2008). Many health professionals accept some of corporate rationalism's tenets, and some become corporate rationalisers themselves, as medical directors in trusts, for example, 'corporate rationalisers from within' (North and Peckham, 2001). Though clinicians' autonomy and power have diminished in some ways, they can still draw on their power to protect their own interests (Salter, 2004). They have sometimes been willing to sacrifice patients' interests to corporate rationalism (Salter, 2004; Chapter Ten).

Corporate rationalism is inimical to clinicians' autonomy, their freedom to treat patients without coercion or interference from other people. That affects patients' autonomy, since if their clinicians are not free to offer them all relevant courses of action or treatments, patients cannot make choices unconstrained by coercion. Clinicians, and therefore patients, are losing autonomy of action, in any case, due to increasingly complex medical technologies, team working and rising costs (Schneider, 1998). How the autonomy of patients can be safeguarded when professionals' autonomy is increasingly restricted is as yet an unexplored issue. It is ironic that, just when patient activists, and some health professionals, have succeeded in gaining some support for patients' autonomy, it could be reduced again through the rise of corporate rationalism.

Whatever interests corporate rationalisers support or deny, their power is now sometimes so great that they, too, can be said to hold dominant interests. The dynamics of the interplay of interests between clinicians and corporate rationalisers are complex. Corporate rationalisers usually have to work through clinicians; and the exact balance of power between them may make no practical difference to what patients experience or do not experience. When, from now on, I refer to dominance and dominant interest holders, I shall not always distinguish between clinicians' dominance and corporate rationalisers' dominance. Dominance is dominance. Behind the curtains at the windows of the GP's surgery and round the beds in the hospital ward stands the shadowy figure of the corporate rationaliser.

Repressed interests and patients

Alford called his third group of interests 'repressed'. Repressed interests were held by the 'community' (Alford, 1975). Alford's 'community' were the American uninsured poor who had no or little healthcare.

In the UK, with a National Health Service that aims to give care to everyone who needs it, this translates into patients and potential patients in the community (Ham, 1981; Williamson, 1988). To be *repressed* is to be checked or restrained in advance, to be prevented from speaking or acting (Little et al, 1936). Repressed interests, Alford said, were not served by social or political structures (Alford, 1975). In the US, as in the UK, social structures that could promote or support patients' interests were sparse in the 1960s. Patients had started to form patient groups, but there were few people who could speak for patients' interests; and those few were easily cooptated by more powerful interest holders (Alford, 1975). Repressed interests could only be served when their holders 'mobilised extraordinary political energies' (Alford, 1975, p 14).

Alford called the few people who could speak for patients' interests 'equal healthcare advocates'. They sought high-quality, accessible, equitable care for everyone (Alford, 1975). Their UK equivalents are called patient representatives or advocates or, more recently, patient activists (Chapter Seven). Although in the 2000s there are more people who can speak for patients' interests than there were in the 1960s, both in the US and in the UK, they and patients still face difficulties.

The consequences of repression

Starting from Alford's framework, we can look at repression in greater detail than he did. There are at least three major ways in which patients' interests can be said to be repressed: (1) through withholding information from patients so that they cannot identify and articulate their interests; (2) through lack of social and political arrangements that could articulate and promote patients' interests effectively; and (3) through unwillingness or refusal to listen to or act on what patients and patient activists say.

1. Withholding of information

Information that patients need to judge whether decisions or courses of action would be in their interests or against their interests is sometimes withheld from them. The withholding may be inadvertent or deliberate. It may be done by professionals or by corporate rationalisers. Not telling parents at Alder Hey and Bristol about the possible retention of their children's organs was an example. Preventing patients or relatives, as in those instances, from having relevant information is coercive. It affronts their autonomy. It prevents them from acting as moral agents, with responsibilities for themselves, their families and all the other people, known and unknown, to whom they are connected in various ways. Repressing patients' interests by withholding information is like trying them in a secret court, without the patients even knowing that they are on trial, and so without giving them an opportunity to defend their interests. It is unjust and leads to other injustices.

2. Lack of social and political arrangements

Patients collectively lack social and political arrangements or structures to help them identify and explain how some of the healthcare they experience, or are denied, affects their interests, as they define those interests, or would define them if they knew they were threatened. Simple resources for patient groups and for individual activists, like money to commission research or to pay for travel to meetings or to subscribe to journals, are scant. This is large-scale, but only partly deliberate, institutionalised repression of patients' interests.

◊◊ One indicator of support for repressed interests would be a national body that could speak for all patients' interests (Alford, 1975). The UK lacks an inclusive, effective national body, though some patient groups have formed alliances with each other (Baggott et al, 2005). Professionals and managers can use their salaries to fund organisations to foster study of their specialty, to promote its influence and to commission research or other projects. Many patient groups are entirely voluntary, so lack money for these purposes. They are reluctant to accept money from the Department of Health or from drug companies, even if it were offered. Some of the work they could do, working for patients' interests, and speaking for them to local and national policy-making and governance bodies, remains undone. ◊◊

3. Unwillingness to listen or to act

Even when patients or patient activists can speak for their own or other patients' interests, corporate rationalisers and professionals are often confused about whom to listen to or how to assess the validity and generality of what they say (Hogg, 2009; Chapters Seven, Eight and Nine). Patient surveys and other ways of eliciting patients' views are common, but generally dominant interest holders retain the choice of what questions to ask (Chapter Five). They can also choose whether to implement changes that could follow from those patients' views (Davies and Cleary, 2005; Reeves and Seccombe, 2008). Patients and patient activists are increasingly invited to take part in consultations by the Department of Health or other official bodies to contribute their views on specific topics and policies (Baggott et al, 2005). On the face of things, they are not prevented from speaking at those meetings. But they may be told that issues they raise are not within the scope of the consultation (Ann Seymour, personal communication, 2002). Moreover, patients' and patient activists' views are seldom readily accepted by dominant interest holders, unless they coincide with their own views (Salter, 2004; Baggott et al, 2005). Conflicts of view do not in themselves indicate dominance and repression. But if one set of participants' views are regularly overridden or ignored, the other participants' de facto dominance supports repression.

The effects of the repression of patients' interests are subtle and far reaching:

1. Repression hinders the identification and discussion of patients' interests by all interest holders, including by patients themselves. Oppressed groups have latent interests, interests that they have not yet put into words (Wrong, 1979). Repression slows down patients' identification of their latent interests, but it does not totally prevent it. If it did, the patient movement could not have come into being. (The identification of latent interests is like 'consciousness raising' in recognised emancipation movements.)

2. It hinders clinicians and corporate rationalisers from understanding the effects of their actions on patients.

    ◊◊ We judge ourselves by our intentions and judge others by the effects of their actions on us, noted Philip Rhodes, explaining why he and his fellow obstetricians saw themselves as kind, compassionate and communicating well, while many of the women they cared for judged them and their invasive tests and procedures brutal (Anon, 1982). ◊◊

Here doctors were aware of how their patients saw them and their actions. But sometimes doctors are unaware, for repression inhibits them from asking certain questions and so prevents patients from responding.

3. It makes it easy for dominant interest holders to assume that actions that suit their interests are also in patients' interests.

◊◊ A group of GPs at a national meeting were congratulating themselves on the referral system in the UK, whereby patients must be referred to a hospital specialist by the GP; they cannot usually refer themselves directly. The GPs took it as an article of faith that this was in patients' interests. They did not consider how the system benefited their own interests in sustaining society's need for GPs and in sustaining their power; or how it benefited the government's interests, in controlling patients via their GPs. They seemed unaware that some patients in this country would prefer to refer themselves directly to specialists (personal observation, 1997). ◊◊

One of the advantages of Alford's way of looking at interests in healthcare is that his concepts of structural interests and of repression imply that dominant interest holders do not necessarily consciously act repressively. The ill consequences of repression are not necessarily intended, nor foreseen. Most health professionals and corporate rationalisers act from motives that are good (Chapter One).

Having set the political scene through Alford's theoretical framework, I now turn to looking more closely at dominance, repression, oppression and coercion, and how they affect patients' interests

Domination

Human tendencies towards domination probably originate in our evolutionary past, for non-human primates and other social animals have systems of dominance and subordination (Wilson, 1975). Dominance, the almost unchecked exercise of power, suits the dominant, though in human societies it can bring with it responsibilities for the basic welfare of the subordinates.

◊◊ Men in 18th- and 19th-century Britain were expected to provide for their wives and unmarried daughters and sisters. ◊◊

Being subordinate can have advantages for non-human primates (Wilson, 1975). It also can for humans. For patients, being excused from certain responsibilities, and being dependent upon people with special expertise, can be a relief from the anguishes and anxieties of serious disease.

◊◊ 'I wish to abdicate all responsibility for my disease to someone who actually understands the nuances of my case', wrote a doctor in training, diagnosed with lymphoma (Ross, 2009, p 21). She meant responsibility for understanding the nature of her disease, her clinical situation and what treatments would be best for her. ◊◊

Dr Nicki Ross was a patient in a privileged position, for doctors are especially well looked after by other doctors (Armstrong, 2009). But the feelings she expressed may be common in patients with serious, potentially fatal, diseases. They may be common, too, in patients who are critically ill but will probably recover, if given expert care. Very ill or weak patients do not necessarily want to be told about their dangerous clinical state or to negotiate with their doctors.

◊◊ David Rier, a medical sociologist who was a patient in an intensive care unit for some weeks, thought that being in a 'cocoon of optimism' had helped to save his life (Rier, 2000, p 79). ◊◊

But:

◊◊ A patient in an ordinary, not a privileged, position, Mitzi Blennerhassett, who, like Nicki Ross, had potentially fatal cancer, felt anguish when her requests for information were refused or fudged (Blennerhassett, 2008). The treatments were necessarily unpleasant and risky; but it was the harshness and deceitfulness of her care, its coercive oppressiveness, that affected her deeply and lastingly (Blennerhassett, 2008). ◊◊

Exactly which responsibilities patients wish to relinquish, when, for what, and on whom they wish to be dependent, varies. The boundary between responsibilities willingly relinquished by patients and responsibilities taken coercively from them is crucial for patients' experiences of their care. It is crucial also for any theory of emancipation.

Coercion, repression and oppression

Dominant interest holders can use their dominant power to support and promote the interests of less powerful interest holders, or to deny and undermine them (Lukes, 2005). They can behave in liberating ways towards other social groups. Or they can behave coercively towards less powerful interest holders (Lukes, 2005). Another distinguished social scientist, Pierre Bourdieu, said that dominant interest holders, both as groups and as individuals, tend to be coercive towards less powerful interest holders (Bourdieu, 1998). *Coercion* primarily means constraining, restraining or compelling by force (Little et al, 1936). But since the 19th century, it has also meant the moral coercion of power-holders' opinions (Chapter One). Some healthcare, like the compulsory detention in hospital of some mentally ill patients, is coercive in an obvious sense. Detained patients cannot leave the hospital without permission. But when healthcare is compulsory, it is subject to legal oversight and patients can appeal against it (Williamson, 2005). For most patients, moral and social coercion is what matters; and much of it is unrecognised in daily patient care.

Dominant interest holders' tendency to coerciveness is supported by, or perhaps even largely caused by, the social structures producing the social status quo and the culture of a particular profession (Bourdieu, 1998). Or dominant interest holders may feel dominated themselves (Bourdieu, 1998).

> ◊◊ Clinicians may feel they are dominated or constrained by corporate rationalisers, corporate rationalisers by clinicians. Their gloomy talk at conferences and in hospital corridors sometimes suggests that each set of interest holders feels helplessly dominated by the other (personal observations, 2007). ◊◊

Social scientists debate how far people's behaviour is directed and constrained by social structures and how far people are free to act as they choose (Sharrock and Watson, 1995). At the same time, social structures also make it possible for people to take action (Sharrock and Watson, 1995). As with other dichotomised pairs, like inheritance or environment, nature or nurture, constraint and freedom interact with each other. Dominant interest holders can sometimes break out of the constraints that seem to bind them.

> ◊◊ Secrecy about what happened at post-mortems at Alder Hey and Bristol was an 'institutionalised condition'. The doctors who practised secrecy had not personally introduced the practice and its standard, 'do not tell relatives or the public'; it was what they had been taught (Bristol Royal Infirmary Inquiry, 2000). Any one of them, however, could have opposed it; institutionalisation seldom totally extinguishes personal responsibility and freedom. One pathologist at Bristol, Professor P.J. Berry, did begin to question the standard and raised it with his surgical colleagues,

who dismissed his concerns (Bristol Royal Infirmary Inquiry, 2000). Unfortunately, he did not raise his doubts with lay people or with patient activists. ◊◊

In addition, however, to structural or institutionalised pressures for coercive policies, practices and standards, dominant interest holders can have personal and deliberate reasons for behaving coercively. They may feel that they are exerting legitimate social control over patients (Chapter Four); or put the need for training future doctors above that for giving a good service to the patients in front of them; or behave coercively for their own convenience; or think that they know what is best for the patient. Shortages of time or other resources will tend to reinforce coercive behaviour, by necessitating or by excusing it.

Conversely, dominant interest holders have the power to behave towards patients in liberating ways. But if they do, and if they go 'too far', they are liable to incur the disapproval of their peers (Chapter Nine).

◊◊ "What you and I are trying to do will take years off our lives," said a consultant in genitourinary medicine to me in 1990. ◊◊

Institutionalised coercion may be overt, open, or covert, hidden. Overt coercion can be experienced as oppression, if patients see no justification for it or deem it against their interests. To be *oppressed* means to be pressed down on, crushed, kept under by the tyrannical use of power (Little et al, 1936). Oppression is closely related to repression, for to be *repressed* means being checked, prevented in advance from acting or speaking (Little et al, 1936). The meanings overlap, but to keep the distinction, I shall use repression when referring to patients' interests, as Alford did, and oppression when referring to patients' experiences. Healthcare can be said to be repressive if patients are unaware that their interests are threatened or denied. Healthcare can be said to be oppressive if patients are aware that their interests are threatened, undermined or denied. The repression of patients' interests paves the way for oppression.

Overt coercion

Patients can feel or experience overt coercion as oppression, when it takes place. They may or may not accept it as just the way things are.

◊◊ In Northallerton Maternity Hospital in 1976, care was openly coercive. Babies were kept in a nursery away from their mothers and fed according to a strict schedule. But a midwife confided to me that she secretly slipped hungry babies to their mothers in the night for a feed. ◊◊

Here, mothers as well as midwives knew the policy, though mothers probably only discovered it after their babies' births. Then they could try to enlist a nice midwife's help; or make a fuss; or walk out of hospital (discharge themselves) early. They were not totally helpless, because oppression tends to elicit resistance, at least in some people and some situations (Dalrymple and Burke, 2006).

Overt coercion always potentially works against patients' interests in their own autonomy. Autonomy is variously defined, but broadly means self-determination and freedom from coercion; it is a fundamental value in western society (Jensen and Mooney, 1990). (For a fuller definition, see Chapter Six.) Some overtly coercive policies and practices threaten patients' autonomy but do not deny it, if patients can see alternative courses of action: shall I accept this? or oppose it? or evade it? as in the Northallerton Maternity Hospital example. But overt coercion that comes without warning, perhaps in the middle of a procedure or when the patient cannot resist it, denies their autonomy, since it forces them into submission. (Chapter Four gives examples of the profound effect this can have on patients.)

Covert coercion

Patients can only feel or experience covert coercion as oppressive after they have discovered that it took place.

> ◊◊ The policies for organ retention at Alder Hey and Bristol were examples of covert coercion. ◊◊

Although patients cannot resist covert coercion while it is taking place, instances of it that come to light can cause 'scandal' if they breach 'ordinary' social values.

> ◊◊ Examining patients vaginally, without their knowledge or consent, while they were unconscious from general anaesthesia, was criticised by patient activists in the 1980s (Robinson, 1985; Winkler and Rosenthal, 1988). The issue resurfaced in the *British Medical Journal* in the early 1990s (Bewley, 1992). In 2003, a medical student did a survey of current practice and found that examinations without consent were still taking place (Coldicott

et al, 2003). Examining patients without their implicit or explicit consent is assault (Bewley, 1992). ◊◊

This trajectory, of an issue identified; ignored; re-identified as if it were a new issue, perhaps several times over; then finally acted on, is probably common for protests against dominant ways of doing things. Political energy is necessary to change dominant interest holders' practices and standards (Alford, 1975).

Covert coercion always threatens patients' autonomy, if it leads them to make decisions or to agree to courses of action that they might not have agreed to, had they been aware that their interests could be threatened (Williamson, 2005). This is why secrecy is always potentially covert coercion.

> ◊◊ At the Alder Hey and Bristol inquiries, some parents said that they would not have agreed to a post-mortem if they had been told about the practice of retaining their children's organs. Others said that they would have agreed, for the sake of other children who could benefit from the use of their child's organs in research or teaching. On discovering what had happened, parents said that they 'could not comprehend how the medical profession could conceal the retention of [their children's] organs by omission' (Royal Liverpool Children's Report, 2001, p 360). ◊◊

Here, parents were unaware of the threat to their interests, indeed, unaware that they had an interest to be threatened in what happened to their children's organs after the post-mortem. That some organs might be retained had never occurred to them, so their interests in the policy were latent. Dominant interest holders maintain their dominance partly by setting the agenda through their talk and their actions in such a way that repressed interest holders remain unaware of their interests and of threats to them (Lukes, 2005).

Not strictly secret, but often withheld from patients, are protocols that set out criteria for referral or treatment, or national and local policies about what treatment and care should or should not be offered (Williamson, 2005).

> ◊◊ Guidelines about the use of statins and other drugs; national leaflets that describe and evaluate the choices that women can make for childbirth; local guidelines about the length of pre-operative fasting, are sometimes withheld from patients (Williamson, 2005). Chapter Six gives a detailed analysis of

the implications of withholding national guidelines on blood transfusion. ◊◊

The number of policies, protocols and guidelines that are inadvertently or deliberately withheld from patients is probably very large (Chapter Seven). Withholding denies patients the ethical value of lucidity, the opportunity to know all relevant details about the situation that they find themselves in (Fried, 1974). Lack of lucidity prevents patients from understanding the opportunities, the constraints and the choices that should be made clear to them (Fried, 1974). It denies their autonomy.

Conclusion

Dominance, whoever holds it, tends to lead to the oppression of subordinate social groups. The repression of patients' interests hinders dominant interest holders from recognising that some of their actions are oppressive. Domination easily slips into coercion and brings with it injustice.

How patients have begun to recognise their institutionalised disadvantage and have tried to oppose it, have tried to free themselves and other patients from coercion and to increase their freedom to act autonomously, is the subject of the rest of the book.

THREE

The patient movement

Without intellectual and theoretical underpinnings, no movement can succeed ...

(Carolyn Heilbrun, feminist literary scholar, 1989, p 20)

Introduction

This chapter defines the patient movement and looks briefly at its early history, then at the diversity of today's patient groups and at a radical–non-radical or conservative dimension that influences the positions groups take on various issues in healthcare. It suggests that the radical part of the patient movement is so similar to recognised emancipation movements that the patient movement can be seen as an emancipation movement in itself, albeit an immature one. It defines patient emancipation and discusses why the patient movement has not been seen as an emancipation movement. Social groups who have experienced oppression outside healthcare are probably quicker than more advantaged social groups to recognise oppression in their experiences of healthcare and more likely to found radical patient groups that are recognisably emancipatory.

The patient movement

The many patient groups and individual patient activists who work to improve healthcare, specifically patient care, make up the patient movement. It is a movement based on its members' values rather than on their socioeconomic positions, as were older social movements like the trade unions. For that reason, social scientists call it a new social movement (Offe, 1984; Baggott et al, 2005). Social movements, old or new, arise as responses to aspects of social life, the ways things are done in a society, that some people begin to see as no longer acceptable. They decide that something must be done to change how life is lived (Rowbotham, 2004). If those people and their ideas can mobilise support from even a few other people, they may lead ultimately to the development of a social movement that changes society. Founding a group to take social action is a common first step. Patient groups are the building blocks of the patient movement, and individual patient activists often gain their first experience in one or more patient groups (Williamson, 1998).

The birth of the patient movement

Exactly when a social movement begins is hard to say. The processes that lead to social change may start well before anything much happens (Pierson, 2004). But at least three sorts of almost simultaneous, closely entangled, sets of factors or interconnected social processes contributed to the birth and early survival of patient groups, and hence of the patient movement in the UK.

1. A shift in social values

In the mid 20th century, there was a general shift in social values, weakening people's faith in authority and lessening their deference to experts of all kinds (Sedgwick, 1982). Medicine had risen in prominence and esteem in the late 19th century. The writer Robert Louis Stevenson (1850–94), who was often ill, wrote that doctors were 'the flower of all mankind' (Stevenson, 1887). By the early 20th century, social, economic and political institutions in western countries supported the medical profession's power and dominant interests (Alford, 1975). But as social values shifted, medicine's expertise and authority began to be challenged, along with those of other professions and high-status social groups (Haug and Sussman, 1969).

2. The poor quality of some medical care

People began to realise that much patient care and treatment was poor. We are now accustomed to patients' autobiographical accounts of their experiences. One of the first and best was published in 1959 by the eminent economist John Vaizey. His short account of his physical and psychological suffering, of the cruelty, the sentimentality, the pain and the threats to his sense of selfhood, during almost two years of treatment for osteomyelitis (an infection of the bones and bone marrow) in three hospitals, starting in 1943 when he was 14, became an influential classic (Vaizey, 1959). Other books followed in the 1960s. Erving Goffman's *Asylums*, published in 1961; Gerda Cohen's *What's wrong with hospitals?* in 1964; and Barbara Robb's *Sans everything*, in 1967, described hospitals as places of degradation, deprivation, humiliation, where patients did not count (Cohen, 1964; Robb, 1967; Goffman, 1968). Cohen drew on the criticisms of healthcare by early radical patient groups, like the National Association for the Welfare of Children in Hospital (NAWCH), founded in 1961, for some of the material in her paperback book (Cohen, 1964). So, in less than three years, some patient groups' views were spreading beyond their members.

These books were widely read. They cast doubt on the altruism and dedication of the medical profession and on its claim to act always in patients' interests.

3. Critical sociological research

Also in the 1960s, sociologists began to study healthcare professionals and institutions more critically than they had before (Gabe et al, 2004). Eliot Freidson's *Profession of Medicine*, 1970, and his *Professional Dominance*, 1970, and Terence J. Johnson's *Professions and Power*, 1972, were influential examples. Their observations and analyses helped to create scepticism about doctors' and nurses' practices and motives. Health professionals' motives and feelings also came under scrutiny from psychoanalytically oriented researchers, notably in the work of Isabel Menzies at the Tavistock Institute of Human Relations in London in the late 1950s and early 1960s (Menzies, 1959).

These works were read by the educated public as well as by academics. Some founders and early members of radical patient groups studied them eagerly, searching for explanations of why professional and institutional care was sometimes so inhumane and fell so far below health professionals' claims to act in patients' interests.

Patient groups, the building blocks of the patient movement

A patient group is a set of people with shared goals, a constitution and a system of governance, even if it is just five or six members who meet in someone's sitting room. Patient groups are a subset of the social group patients. In the UK, patient groups started in the late 1950s and early 1960s. Two early radical patient groups, NAWCH and the Association for Improvements in the Maternity Services (AIMS), are described in Chapter Four.

Patient groups are now many and diverse (Wood, 2000; Brown and Zavestoski, 2004; Baggott et al, 2005). Patient groups themselves, social scientists and commentators categorise them in various ways, depending on which aspects of the groups seem to them to be important. Pressure, support, activist, protest, self-help, disease, disability, illness, population-based, formal alliance, are some of the categories favoured (Brown and Zavestoski, 2004; Baggott et al, 2005). (The term 'self-help' is confusing, since it can mean mutual support or support plus pressure to improve some aspects of healthcare. Besides, patient groups aim to benefit other patients, not just themselves.) Most groups combine support for patients with some attempt to influence the provision of care or its standards, but their emphases vary.

Patient groups are also diverse in size of membership; criteria for membership; arrangements for governance; whether health professionals are eligible for membership of the governance body and in what proportion to the patient members; sources of funding; stated objectives; whether national or local or both; what sort of publications they produce; and so on (Wood, 2000; Brown and Zavestoski, 2004, Baggott et al, 2005). Some are led by health professionals, some by professionals and patients in partnership, some by patients (Hogg, 1999).

Amid all this variation, however, there seems to be a constant or universal variable that cuts across all patient groups, however they are categorised. It is a radical–non-radical dimension or variable (Borkman, 1997). Thomasina Borkman said that radical groups saw patients' interests as sometimes compatible with health professionals' interests, sometimes in conflict with them; they examined professionals' views and policies, practices and standards of care critically; they expected to be in conflict with professionals over some issues (Borkman, 1997). Non-radical groups saw patients' and professionals' interests as usually compatible with each other; they saw themselves as complementing professionals' work; they were seldom in conflict with them (Borkman, 1997). Some groups were strongly radical or strongly non-radical; most groups were in between (Borkman, 1997). (Borkman's patient groups were in the US; empirical evidence that this variable holds in the UK is given in Chapter Eight).

This radical–non-radical variable seems to have been little noticed by other social scientists. But it is important for understanding why the patient movement is fragmented (Chapter Eight). It is important also, as we shall see later in this chapter, for deciding what sort of a social movement the patient movement is.

Radical and conservative patient groups

To be radical is to uproot generally accepted assumptions, to see beneath the apparent meanings of things (Little et al, 1936). Non-radical can be called conservative, and I shall use this term, although it is not wholly satisfactory because of its party-political meaning in the UK. To be conservative is to accept the status quo, preserve or keep unchanged existing institutions (Little et al, 1936). Radical challenges to the dominant status quo can be reactionary or regressive, aimed at reducing the freedom of other people or even at destroying their institutions and their lives. Or they can be progressive or liberating, aimed at increasing other people's freedom. What 'radical' implies depends on the context and on the speaker's purpose. I use the term radical to mean progressive or liberating challenges to some aspects of the status quo, and non-radical or conservative to mean acceptance of the status quo.

Since most health professionals are conservative, as dominant interest holders supporting the status quo and supported by it (Chapter Two and see next section), conservative patient groups' views accord or are in alignment with those of most professionals. Conservative groups support dominant interest holders' dominant interests. A secondary meaning of radical is to hold advanced views of political reform on democratic lines (Little et al, 1936). 'Advanced views' tells us that radical groups are probably in a minority, for 'ordinary' views reflect current social norms and values. Most patients and the public (the public are people who are not in clinical relationships at a given time) accept dominant interest holders' interests (Alford, 1975). Another secondary meaning of radical is to support an extreme section of a political party (Brown, 1993). These secondary meanings link radical patient groups, who can seem extreme to conservative groups, to the rest of the patient movement.

Both radical and conservative patient groups work to improve healthcare. Conservative groups see deficiencies in healthcare as largely due to scarcity of resources and, like some professionals, they often press for more resources. They see healthcare as mostly doing good. Radical groups also value the good that healthcare does, and could do, and sometimes press for more resources. But they see also harms to patients and to their interests in healthcare as it exists at any given time, its status quo, that more resources will not necessarily improve.

The actions of radical and conservative patient groups and individual activists

When radical patient groups or individuals question or oppose aspects of the status quo, the policies, practice or standards that most professionals work to, they are opposing dominant interests. They question or oppose coercive practices that could harm patients' interests, as patients define those interests, or would define them, if they knew they might be threatened. They are quick to identify repressive and oppressive policies, practices and standards. They scrutinise new policies and practices, lest they contain coercive elements, implications or consequences. In taking action against the repression of patients' interests or against oppressive, coercive policies, practices and standards, they take emancipatory action.

By contrast, conservative groups, by accepting the status quo and supporting dominant interests, are liable to support oppressive policies and standards. In practice, conservative and radical groups can be hard to tell apart because, except for strongly conservative and strongly radical groups, the positions they take on some issues can overlap or be the same. But some points can be made.

1. Conservative positions supporting the status quo are, politically, default positions. Taking a conservative position on an issue requires no special knowledge, energy or political skill, merely agreement with what dominant interest holders say or do.

   ◊◊ All but two of the non-executive directors of a trust supported the executive directors' recommendation that money should be spent on employing more obstetricians. As business men, none knew much about the maternity services. A health economist and I argued that the money would be better spent on employing more midwives. Our arguments, his for cost-effectiveness, mine for higher quality of care, failed (personal observation, 1996). ◊◊

   To be radical, a group or individual must analyse patients' interests as patients define them, or as they would define them, if they knew they were threatened. Conservative groups and individuals support dominant interest holders' interests by accepting their ideologies and ways of doing things, their policies, practices and standards. Their position is the easier. But sometimes their acceptance may be unconscious, in the sense of not deliberately thought out.

2. Because radical positions require thought and effort, it can sometimes be hard to tell the difference between conservative views that are held from conviction and conservative views that are held because their holder does not know enough about the topic to challenge or oppose the status quo.

3. People may take conservative positions because they align themselves emotionally or pragmatically with health service staff (Williamson, 2008a). Since everyone is likely to need the help of clinicians at some time, or has already benefited from their expert care or their kindness, feelings of gratitude, dependence, prudence or fear tend to make people align themselves with staff, unless something has happened to radicalise them (Chapter Four).

4. Conservatives probably either see coercive elements in policies, practices and standards less readily than radicals do; or they see them as legitimate; or as necessary for staff's morale or convenience (Williamson, 2008a).

These four points are interrelated and are discussed in Chapter Eight.

5. A fifth point relevant to radicalness and conservatism is methodologically and theoretically very important: over time, radical ideas can become conservative. Judging whether a position or an idea is conservative or radical depends on when the judgement is made (Williamson, 2008a). Telling radical and conservative ideas apart at any given time depends on knowing the history of a particular issue and how far and how widely the once-radical position on it has been accepted or rejected. Unless researchers and commentators take this into account and can trace these trajectories accurately, their judgements may be wrong.

   ◊◊ A standard widely accepted both by conservative and by radical groups in the patient movement, that mixed-sex wards are undesirable and should be abolished, may seem new and radical to commentators outside the movement, simply because they have not met it before. ◊◊

Tracing the trajectory of issues and ideas accurately is important because it shows how the status quo, the accepted ways of doing things, can change over time. Yesterday's radical ideas become today's conservative ideas, if and when enough professionals and patient groups come to accept them. This is important theoretically, because, once radical ideas become widely accepted, they are no longer radical. They become so much part of the status quo that people forget they were ever radical and controversial (Williamson, 1999a; Williamson, 2008a).

◊◊ NAWCH's campaign to get children's wards to allow parents to visit their children at any time and for as long as they liked, rather than at restricted times, created anger and resistance in some paediatric staff and took more than 30 years to succeed (Williamson, 1992). Now everyone takes it for granted that, when children are in hospital, parents and children must have free access to each other, day and night. ◊◊

This is how radical ideas become accepted. The whirlpools of agitation that radical ideas create sink back as the river flows on. But the river itself is changed.

My hypothesis that the patient movement is an emancipation movement

All new social movements challenge dominant social and political ways of doing things (Baggott et al, 2005). Can we go further than this generalisation for the patient movement? Can the patient movement, made up as it is of conservative and radical patient groups and individual activists, be said to be an emancipation movement? Can it be said to be an emancipation movement if many of its members, let alone people outside it, do not think of it as such? That is a question touched on in Chapter One.

Emancipation or liberation movements differ from other social movements – anti-nuclear war or green ecology movements, for example – in that their members have personal experience of being oppressed (Mansbridge, 2001a). Almost all patient groups take their authority from their members' personal experience of healthcare (Baggott et al, 2005). Conservative and radical patient groups have that in common. It is how patients perceive and interpret their experiences, and what they do about it, that makes a major difference between radical and conservative patient groups. It is with radical patient groups that any claim of the patient movement to be emancipatory must, in the first place, lie.

The emancipation hypothesis that I put forward for healthcare is this: *the radical parts of the patient movement seek to support patients' autonomy in healthcare, freeing them from coercion and from other harms related to differences in power between patients, professionals and corporate rationalisers.*

They seek to lift repression from patients' interests and oppression from their experiences. Inasmuch as some, perhaps most, of these radical ideas and new emancipatory standards come to be accepted by non-radical patient groups, the patient movement can be called an emancipation movement.

An unrecognised emancipation movement?

That the patient movement is an emancipation movement has been unrecognised, I think, for several reasons.

1. The position of patients is unusual. Patienthood is usually only temporary, even though the consequences of episodes of healthcare, for good or ill, can last a lifetime. Moreover, anyone can become a patient: a health professional or a corporate rationaliser as much as someone unconnected with healthcare. Reciprocally, patients or former patients can, if they are accepted for training, become health professionals or corporate rationalisers. Such interchangeability is rare: men cannot become biological women or white people biological black people.

2. The medical profession's ideological, political and structural dominance is well established and sustained largely because so many people accept it, even if no longer always uncritically. Alford posed the question of whether people give doctors their power because doctors do good and useful work or because doctors' power makes people see their work as good and useful (Alford, 1975). It is probably both, interacting with each other.

   Corporate rationalism's ideological, political and structural position is little understood by patients and the public; and its progress towards new dominance little noticed or challenged yet (Williamson, 2008b).

3. In contrast to dominant interest holders and their institutions, the patient movement has little support from social structures (Chapter Two) and lacks a coherent ideology to guide its members' actions and explain them to people outside it. In 1969, Marie Haug and Marvin Sussman said that patients' resistance to clinical care was generally still incipient (Haug and Sussman, 1969). Forty years later, resistance is no longer always incipient. But the lack of an ideology is the mark of an immature social movement (Mansbridge, 2001b). That lack and that immaturity hinder discussions and analyses both inside and outside the movement.

4. The history of the patient movement is short. It is easy to suppose that well-established emancipation movements, like the women's, the black civil rights, the disabilities rights movements, started out with ideas and ultimate goals clearly thought out and put into words. But probably they seldom, if ever, flew from their nests fully fledged. More likely, they arose as scattered small groups, each with its own immediate purpose (Chapter One). This was how patient groups started in the late 1950s and early 1960s in the UK. Patient groups' purposes and values are diverse (Baggott et al, 2005). Half a century on from the founding of the early radical patient groups, this contributes to the patient movement remaining weak, fragmented and confusing (Williamson, 1999a; Salter, 2003; 2004).

5. Scarcity of resources of all kinds afflicts many patient groups (Chapter Two). In the UK, for example, there is no general journal for patients and patient activists that imparts information, hosts debate and creates feelings of collegiality, the sense of belonging to a unique and special community, as professional journals do.

6. Strongly radical patient groups are probably a small minority of patient groups. Radical groups seem prone to fade away as they achieve some of their goals, or to become less radical (Hogg, 1999). Radical patient activists tend to believe that employing paid staff to cope with heavy workloads of questions and requests from patients also diminishes a group's or an organisation's radicalness. Staff's interests in securing salaries and careers for themselves are not the same as the radical group's founders' interests in going against the status quo of established social structures. In any case, organisations tend to slip away from the intentions of those who first created them (Pierson, 2004).

7. Patient groups' and individual activists' eagerness to have their desired standards accepted, and the readiness of some professionals to accept and claim them for themselves, obscures the impact and successes of patient activists' ideas and work (Chapter Ten). Dominant interest holders' readiness to claim activists' ideas means that resistance to radical or emancipatory ideas may seem less intractable in healthcare than elsewhere. Though this is welcome, it may make the boundary between patients, as repressed interest holders, and professionals and corporate rationalisers, as dominant interest holders, ambiguous or faint.

8. Conversely, activists take and promote some ideas from health professionals (Chapter Ten). This again blurs the boundary.

9. Radical patient activists take actions that are emancipatory; but they do not necessarily see them as such. This is largely because they seldom tie them in to the theoretical terms that social and political scientists use in discussing power, dominance, oppression, repression, inequality, injustice (Chapter Two).

◊◊ To my question, "When did a theoretical or ideological perspective begin to clarify in your mind?" one radical activist replied, "When I did a PhD [in social science]" (personal communication, 2006). ◊◊

Steps towards recognition?

Radical patient groups usually start from the personal level of their own members' experiences of healthcare; then move on to interpreting these experiences through a middle level, marked by words like 'oppression'; then move their focus to a high level, marked by comparisons with other oppressed groups, emancipation movements and mention of structural factors (Crossley and Crossley, 2001; Edwards, 2005). The personal becomes the political, and the political becomes the personal, as in recognised emancipation movements (Sherwin, 1992).

This progression takes place most quickly, I suggest, in social groups that have already experienced oppression or discrimination outside healthcare: people with severe, irreversible physical disabilities, people who have chronic or recurrent mental illness, and people who are female, among others. These social groups have recognised emancipatory or liberation movements (Rogers and Pilgrim, 1991; Crossley and Crossley, 2001; Groch, 2001; Mansbridge and Morris, 2001; Thomas, 2007). Members of these social groups are accustomed to discerning oppression. Moreover, when they become patients, they may meet difficulties and disadvantages over and above those met by patients who come to patienthood from more fortunate social groups. There are at least three aspects of healthcare that they may find discriminatory or in some other way repressive or oppressive.

First, treatments specifically related to the illnesses, impairments or conditions that led to their oppression in the first place are likely to be more problematic and controversial than treatments for illnesses from which anyone can suffer. Many clinical treatments could probably be improved or superseded. Many clinicians are likely to prefer some treatments over others. But psychiatry, obstetrics and gynaecology and some parts of neurology are conspicuously controversial. They are controversial in part because, in them, social and medical models of illness and disability tend to be jumbled up. (Social models of illness attribute illness and impairment to social factors; medical models to biological factors.) The two sets of factors interact; but which one individual patients and professionals consider more important in any given clinical or institutional situation varies.

◊◊ Patients with depression are not always offered a choice between behavioural therapies or electroconvulsive therapy (ECT). ECT is a controversial treatment, thankfully embraced by some patients and psychiatrists, fearfully shunned by others (Webber, 2009). ◊◊

◊◊ Major surgical operations relevant only to women, like hysterectomies and caesarean sections, are controversial because the reasons for which they should be performed are disputed and the rates at which they are performed are rising (Yeo, 1990). Some women feel that such treatments are too harsh or too interventionist and show that clinicians are indifferent to their long-term welfare as women (Campaign Against Hysterectomy and Unnecessary Operations on Women, 1997). Others find these treatments helpful. ◊◊

Second, for treatments for diseases and conditions common to all patients, members of disadvantaged groups may be treated less effectively than members of more advantaged social groups.

◊◊ That women receive less often than men treatments from which both could benefit has been shown repeatedly (Sharp, 1998). Men and women with end-stage renal disease in the US are equally likely to receive kidney transplants up to the age of 45 (Tanne, 2009). After that age, women are less likely to receive transplants than men with the same health status, even though they would benefit as much as or more than men (Tanne, 2009). ◊◊

Third, members of disadvantaged social groups are accustomed to being spoken to in patronising or demeaning ways. Women, for example, are often addressed as "love" while men nearby are "sir". Disadvantaged patients may meet with similar affronts in hospitals and GPs' surgeries, just as all patients may. But they may meet them in stronger form.

◊◊ A former user of mental health services described 'being patronised, insulted and invalidated by health [service] staff' (Brotchie and Wann, 1993, p 9). ◊◊

Points like these suggest that patients from oppressed social groups might be more sensitive to poor care, or to the possibility of poor care, than other patients. They might be more radical in opposing it and more likely to found radical patient groups. The case of women suggests that these points hold good. Women are less likely to be satisfied with their healthcare than men.

◊◊ Eight per cent of women were dissatisfied with primary care, while only 2% of men were (Calnan and Williams, 1990). ◊◊

◊◊ Women rated their experience of care for stroke significantly more negatively than did men (Healthcare Commission, 2005). ◊◊

◊◊ Women were more likely than men to complain about medical mishaps and accidents (Fallberg and Calltorp, 1999). ◊◊

Probably, more women than men found radical patient groups. That women are preponderant in radical patient groups and as individual radical patient activists is a generally held impression that has never been satisfactorily explained. The six radical patient groups in Chapter Four happen to fit this impression. Of two prompted by concerns about the treatment of patients of both sexes, one was founded by a group of men and women, the other by a woman. The other four were, at first sight, predominantly about women's concerns and were founded by women. But one benefited fathers as well as mothers, and children of both sexes; another, the partners of women in childbirth as well as the women, and baby boys as much as baby girls; the other two raised issues about radiotherapy and about research that were as relevant to men patients as to women patients. So, apart from sex-specific diseases like ovarian or prostate cancer, there are no strict boundaries between men and women as beneficiaries of patient groups.

A few radical patient groups explicitly connect their oppression as women to their oppression as patients. From its early days, AIMS, founded in 1960, for example, described much maternity care as oppressive, and still does (Edwards, 2005). AIMS consciously took, and takes, a liberating stance (Edwards, 2005). But many radical patient groups, working for both men and women patients, do not see their actions as liberating or emancipatory.

Just as radical patient groups take emancipatory actions without necessarily defining them as such, researchers and commentators also sometimes describe patient groups that challenge medical policy, beliefs, research and practice, without calling those groups emancipatory. (Brown and Zavestoski's paper is an example, Brown and Zavestoski, 2004). Yet some of those groups challenge dominant coercive policies and practices and work to change policies and standards in directions that support patients' autonomy, just as recognised emancipation movements do (Williamson, 2007a; 2008a).

Similarly, health professionals and policy analysts occasionally use the word emancipatory in referring to specific policies or practices that support patients' autonomy, without applying the idea more widely. (Examples are Grol, 1999; Allsop et al, 2004; Mol, 2008.)

Most surprisingly of all, people have often remarked on parallels between the patient movement and the women's and civil rights movements (Rogers and Pilgrim, 1991; Sherwin, 1992; Williamson, 1999a; Crossley and Crossley, 2001). But even with these parallels, a view of the patient movement as an emancipation movement seems not to have emerged.

Comment

If the patient movement comes to be seen as an emancipation movement, the way we look at healthcare will change. It could change in constructive ways, enabling clinicians, corporate rationalisers and patients to work together for higher standards of care and for a health service that does justice to its providers' good intentions. Chapter Eleven returns to these thoughts.

FOUR

Radicalisation

... every general principle brings with it, by the insight which it furnishes, disillusionment as well as elucidation ... elucidation, in that it enables us to see everywhere throughout the most complicated relations the same simple facts.

(Ernst Mach, physicist and philosopher, 1883, p 88)

Introduction

This chapter looks at the founding of six radical patient groups between 1960 and 1998, as recounted in their founders' own words, and at the radicalisation of two individual radical patient activists. The groups and individuals were a convenience sample of groups and individuals whom I knew to be strongly radical. All challenged the status quo of dominant interest holders' ways of doing things, their practices and standards. All challenged them in the direction of increasing patients' freedom from coercion and freedom to choose how to act. From these eight accounts, we can see that the conditions that social scientists postulate are necessary to radicalise members of oppressed social groups applied here for patients receiving everyday healthcare, like women having babies, patients having radiotherapy, patients taking prescribed medicines. These radicalised patients 'awoke' to political or 'oppositional' consciousness, just as members of recognised emancipation movements do.

The conditions necessary for radicalisation

Social scientists believe that three conditions are necessary for what they call awakening to (or the birth of) political or oppositional consciousness in recognised emancipation movements and I, referring to the patient movement, call radicalisation:

- A perception of harm
- A perception of indignity or injustice

- A sense of social efficacy (Klandermans, 1997; Goodwin et al, 2001; Mansbridge and Morris, 2001).

In the accounts that follow, we can look for these three conditions.

The radical patient groups and individual activists

The six patient groups were the Association for Improvements in the Maternity Services, the National Association for the Welfare of Children in Hospital, the Bristol Survey Support Group, the Radiotherapy Action Group Exposure, the Insulin Dependent Diabetic Trust and the Adverse Psychiatric Reactions Information Link. The individual activists were Jean Robinson and Mitzi Blennerhassett, each eminent in her own field of patient activism. The groups were diverse in the issues they identified and addressed; in the sizes of their membership; and in how long they flourished. All were national voluntary organisations in the UK. One employed a few paid staff; in the others, all work was unpaid. Five of the founders of groups and both the individual activists have written their own accounts of their early days. A sixth account was written by commentators drawing on Radiotherapy Action Group Exposure members' accounts.

AIMS Association for Improvements in the Maternity Services

Founded 1960, challenges psychosocial and clinical care.

Complaints about impersonal care, lack of information, long waiting times in antenatal clinics, and healthcare professionals' continual focus on the abnormal in maternity care have been recorded since 1915 (Tew, 1990). Patient groups aiming to improve maternity care started in the late 1950s. Of these groups, AIMS has consistently been the most radical.

Sally Willington founded the Society for the Prevention of Cruelty to Pregnant Women, later changed to the Association for Improvements in the Maternity Services, AIMS, in 1960, after she had experienced six weeks of care in a maternity hospital. In a letter to *The Observer*, 1 April 1960, she wrote: 'In hospital, as a matter of course presumably, mothers put up with loneliness, lack of sympathy, lack of privacy, lack of consideration, poor food, unlikely visiting hours, callousness, regimentation, lack of instruction, lack of rest, deprivation of the new baby, stupidly rigid routines, rudeness, a complete disregard of mental care or the personality of the mother.' She invited readers who thought that 'something should be done' to write to her and join the Society. Other mothers joined and local groups sprang up all over Britain (Willington, 2007).

AIMS constantly keeps under review and opposes much obstetric policy, practice and research. It argues that many routine practices, that is, practices that are compulsory, unless the woman successfully refuses them, can harm mothers and babies, physically by episiotomy, for example; physiologically by induction of the baby's birth, for example; and psychologically by reducing labouring women's confidence and self-esteem or by disrupting mother–baby bonding. AIMS has contributed so successfully to ridding maternity care of some practices, like enemas and pubic shaves in early labour and the sequestration of healthy newborn babies in nurseries, that many people are scarcely aware that these practices ever existed in the UK. AIMS continues to campaign for better maternity care, keeping pace with new issues and problems, as they arise, and persisting with old, unresolved issues.

AIMS' current stated objectives are 'Working towards normal birth; providing independent support and information about maternity choices; raising awareness of current research on childbirth and related issues' (www.aims.org.uk). 'Working towards normal birth' means trying to ensure that obstetric interventions are used only when the clinical condition of a mother or foetus justify them, not routinely. AIMS sees pregnancy and childbirth as natural biological processes: obstetricians see them as medical processes (Graham and Oakley, 1989).

AIMS is wholly voluntary (unpaid), with a national committee of 8–10 members and four regional networks. It currently has 871 individual members and 117 organisation or group members (Glenys Rowlands, membership secretary, personal communication, 2008).

NAWCH National Association for the Welfare of Children in Hospital

Founded 1961, challenges psychosocial care.

Hospitals in the UK are descended from charitable and poor law institutions (Cohen, 1964). Those institutions separated members of families; and this tradition remains in force. Even today, many hospitals impose severely restricted visiting times on their adult patients.

In 1961, in a series of articles in *The Observer* Sunday newspaper, and on television, James Robertson, from the Tavistock Institute of Human Relations in London, argued that children in hospital, especially young children, should not to be separated from their mothers (Robertson, 1961). He urged people to press for the implementation of the Ministry of Health's policies for children in hospital, based on a report that the government had accepted, the Platt Report of 1959 (Robertson, 1961; Ministry of Health, 1959). Peg Belson, Jane Thomas and a few friends, other mothers living in Battersea, London, took up the challenge and founded Mother Care for Children in Hospital, later changed to the National Association for the Welfare of Children in Hospital, in 1961, under Robertson's guidance (Belson, 1981; 2004). Though none of their own children had been in hospital, these mothers were deeply affected by accounts of the plight of children separated from their mothers, portrayed in James Robertson's film, *A two-year-old goes to hospital*, and book, *Young children in hospital* (Robertson, 1953; 1958). These mothers, and others who joined NAWCH, believed that separations could have long-term harmful psychological and developmental consequences for the child, and sometimes harmful physical consequences. The story of Dawn, a child just 3 years old, who cried inconsolably for her mother and haemorrhaged to death after a tonsillectomy in 1965, was published in *The Lancet* and widely circulated to NAWCH members (Hales-Tooke, 1973).

It took almost 30 years of effort by national and local NAWCH members, meeting paediatricians, civil servants and managers, getting questions asked of ministers in the House of Commons, putting on conferences and conducting surveys, before unrestricted visiting was accepted in all children's wards in the UK (Williamson, 1992). Like AIMS, NAWCH took up many other issues; but unlike AIMS, it took up mainly psychosocial ones.

By 1962, there were 30 local NAWCH branches, by 1975, 53 (Hales-Tooke, 1973; Belson, 2004). NAWCH developed into an influential organisation, with mixed lay and professional membership and trustees, employing paid staff nationally and three regional development officers. In 1988, NAWCH played a major part in establishing EACH, the European Association for Children in Hospital. This now has 20 member countries and a charter, first published in 1984, based on the British NAWCH charter (EACH, 2002).

As the situation for children in hospital improved and unrestricted visiting became accepted, NAWCH gradually became less radical. It changed its name to Action for Sick Children in 1993 and now has six groups (branches) and a small office (Peg Belson, personal communication, 2009). While, in general, the care of sick children has improved, clinical and ethical issues remain. Moreover, some children and adolescents are still admitted to adult wards, cared for by staff not necessarily trained to take account of their social and emotional needs.

BSSG Bristol Survey Support Group

Founded 1990, challenged clinical research.

Orthodox medicine is suspicious of complementary medicine, but some patients find it helpful. In 1986 two major cancer charities funded a trial to compare the survival and quality of life of women who had received complementary therapy for breast cancer in addition to orthodox treatment, with those of women who had received orthodox treatment only (Goodare, 1996a).

The research was to be a 5-year study of 334 women who had received both orthodox and complementary therapy and 451 women who had received orthodox therapy only. The women in the complementary therapy arm of the trial, given at the Bristol Cancer Help Centre, filled in annual questionnaires about their welfare. The women in the orthodox or control arm of the trial had been enrolled in the trial without their knowledge or consent, from their medical records, and so filled in no questionnaires. The research team published interim findings after only two years, while the women in the complementary arm of the trial were still filling in the latest questionnaire. The findings appeared to show that women in the complementary arm tripled their chances of metastatic spread and doubled their chances of dying (Goodare, 1996a). Goodare, as a patient in the trial, realised that something was wrong. She and another patient, Isla Bourke, founded the BSSG to challenge the scientific and statistical methodology and therefore the validity of the research (Goodare, 1996a). Twenty-three women joined the patient group.

Immediately on its publication, the study was also severely criticised by statisticians and some doctors (Goodare, 1996a). BSSG's and others' criticisms discredited the research and its findings. But the cancer charities had already publicised the findings widely (Goodare, 1996a).

The members of BSSG thought that they should have been told of the interim findings before they were published; that cancer charities should have checked the findings before publicising them; and that, when the research became discredited, the researchers should have apologised to them. The women felt 'first incredulity, and then profound anger'; they felt they had been used as pawns (Goodare, 1996a, p 1; Goodare, 1996c).

Heather Goodare had other distressing experiences, like being treated as a child when she asked her oncologist about the side effects of the anti-oestrogen tamoxifen and was told there were none. (She knew that all drugs can have side effects.) After taking tamoxifen, she found that her singing voice had been damaged. She also discovered that her type of tumour had not been oestrogen-dependent and so could not have benefited from tamoxifen. 'Willy nilly I have become an activist' (Goodare, 1996b, p 128).

BSSG stopped active work after the Charities Commission, to whom BSSG had complained, reprimanded the cancer charities for their uncritical publicising of the trial's findings. Goodare went on to chair the research committee of the UK Breast Cancer Coalition, then to found a more radical break-away patient group, Breast UK (Breast-cancer Research Ethics and Advocacy Strategy UK). Breast UK members kept clinical research for breast cancer under surveillance, criticising research protocols, requesting meetings with researchers and speaking at international conferences. In 2003 the group changed its name to Breast Cancer UK, changing focus to become more active in seeking out the causes of breast cancer and campaigning for a greater emphasis on environmental factors in aetiology. It has six trustees, most of whom have been treated for recurrent breast cancer, and nearly 700 supporters (Clare Dimmer, personal communication, 2008; www.breastcanceruk.org.uk).

RAGE Radiotherapy Action Group Exposure

Founded 1991, challenges clinical care: radiotherapy.

That radiation could kill cancer cells, leaving normal cells relatively unharmed, has been known for more than a century (Munro, 2007). In the 1920s it was discovered that radiation treatment could be made less damaging to normal tissue if the total dose were split into fractions, with treatments given on several days instead of in one treatment (Rodger, 1998). In 1966 a first key paper on radiation-induced irreversible damage to nerves in the brachial plexus (a network of nerves that pass from the spinal cord through the armpit to the arm) was published in the *British Medical Journal* and followed by many other papers to the same effect (Sikora, 1994). During the 1970s and 1980s, however, oncologists used widely different fractionation regimes and techniques for treating breast cancer, based largely upon their own preferences (Sikora, 1994).

Jan Millington and Audrey Ironside founded RAGE in 1991, when they and other women found damage to their bodies some years after they had been treated for breast cancer by radiotherapy, and after their doctors had denied any possible connection between the two (Hanley and Staley, 2006). Publicity in the press about the case of Audrey Ironside, who unsuccessfully tried to sue her radiologist and hospital for medical negligence, alerted other women to injuries they had in common and to their probable cause (Hanley and Staley, 2006).

The women who came forward to RAGE were angry at not having been forewarned of the risks of treatment, nor given any explanation about their injuries after they had occurred. The injuries were serious, including constant pain and progressive loss of the use of their arm; brittle bones; and damage to the heart, lungs, skin and gut. All were thought to be untreatable and some ended in death (Hanley and Staley, 2006). Even after their doctors knew that their patients were suffering from radiation damage, some continued to deny to them 'that there was any problem at all' (RAGE member A, in Hanley and Staley, 2006, p 16). Telling her consultant about her increasing pain and disablement led to RAGE member C being 'treated as if I were a troublemaker' (Hanley and Staley, 2006, p 20).

RAGE aims 'to campaign for national standards in radiotherapy; to raise awareness of the injuries and campaign for sympathetic medical care; to seek compensation commensurate with the injury; and to provide mutual support' (Hanley and Staley, 2006). RAGE has failed to gain government money for each woman injured that would enable her to buy practical help or complementary therapies that might help her disability and pain. But it has succeeded in raising radiologists' understanding of the risks of radiotherapy and in improving its application (Hanley and Staley, 2006).

Radiation damage is still appearing years after radiologists were alerted through the Royal College of Radiologists to the need for care with fractionation regimes and with the positions patients were put in to receive radiation (RAGE Editorial, 2007). An article in the *Daily Mail*, 10 July 2007, resulted in a 'staggering' number of telephone calls to Jan Millington and many new members (RAGE, 2007). Patients were still not being told that 'certain injuries were possible and, should they occur, would be permanent, severe and incurable, even if doctors believed them to be rare …' (RAGE, 2007).

RAGE has a national committee of voluntary members. At the height of its work and publicity, it had 600 members (Jan Millington, personal communication, 2008).

IDDT Insulin Dependent Diabetic Trust

Founded in 1994, challenges clinical care: the prescription of insulins.

In the early 1920s, it was discovered that insulin extracted from slaughtered cattle or pigs could control the levels of glucose in the blood of patients whose pancreases did not produce this complex hormone

(British Medical Association and Royal Pharmaceutical Society of Great Britain, 2004). In 1982 synthetic 'human' insulin, insulin of rDNA origin, became available and began to be prescribed (Hirst, 1997/98). By 1985 patients began to complain of its side effects (Hirst, 1997/98).

In 1994 Jenny Hirst, whose daughter had diabetes, and Dr Matt Kiln, a GP with diabetes, with three other 'angry people', two other men and another woman, founded IDDT as a break-away group from a major diabetes charity, the British Diabetic Association (BDA), now Diabetes UK (Hirst, 1997/98). Hirst, a trustee of the BDA, discovered that pharmaceutical companies, with the agreement of the doctor-dominated BDA national committee, wanted to replace animal insulin entirely with the more profitable synthetic insulin (Hirst, 1997/98). Hirst's daughter had suffered adverse effects from synthetic insulin, similar to those reported in almost 3,000 letters to the BDA from patients or their relatives between 1986 and 1989. Some patients found that, compared with animal insulin, synthetic insulin gave more erratic control of blood sugar levels and had distressing side effects, including gain in weight, pain in joints and muscles, depression and general debilitation. It was less safe for some patients because it gave no warning of imminent hypoglycaemic attacks, which led to comas. Occasional deaths of healthy young people resulted, the 'dead in bed' syndrome (Hirst, 2003). Moreover, patients' medication had often been changed from animal to synthetic insulin without notice. When patients complained, neither their own doctors nor those of the DBA believed their accounts. 'We all experienced being dismissed as neurotic or extremist with some sort of axe to grind ...' (Hirst, 2004, p 1). Some patients were even sent to psychologists or psychiatrists (Hirst, 1997/98). After 'a hard fought battle within the BDA between people with diabetes and the medical establishment', a sociologist was commissioned to analyse a sample of the 3,000 letters sent to the BDA (Hirst, 1997/98, p 5). The report from that study was never published. At that point, Hirst resigned from the BDA and set up IDDT (Hirst, 1997/98; 2004).

IDDT presses for 'Provision of evidence of risks and benefits of ALL treatment options and this evidence must be from *independent* high quality research uninfluenced by the pharmaceutical industry' and 'Commitment to the provision of knowledge and information about ALL treatment options and an undertaking that patients' views will carry equal weight in decision-making about their treatment' (IDDT, 2006, p 626).

IDDT supposes that it is seen as 'the naughty child', the 'non-compliant patient organisation' among other patient organisations for diabetes, because it alone is independent and uninfluenced by the pharmaceutical industry or its funds (Hirst, 2005b, p 1). Its belief that synthetic insulin had no advantages over animal insulin was supported by a review by the independent Cochrane Centre in 2002 (Hirst, 2002). But doctors and diabetes nurse specialists have continued to prescribe synthetic insulin and the threat that animal insulin will be withdrawn remains.

IDDT has a national committee of voluntary members and trustees. It is now an international umbrella organisation with 5,000 members, people living with diabetes, in countries throughout the world, including Canada, the US, Australia and India (Jenny Hirst, personal communication, 2008).

APRIL Adverse Psychiatric Reactions Information Link

Founded in 1998, challenges clinical and regulatory care: the regulation and prescription of drugs.

Controlling what medicines are available in the UK and what information about them must be provided for patients is the task of the statutory Medicines and Healthcare products Regulation Agency (MHRA) (2004). It licenses medicines and places conditions on their prescription and sales and on the information that must be supplied in written form to patients with each packet of medicine. It keeps medicines under surveillance for adverse drug reactions (unwanted side effects or complications) after the medicines are licensed and are being taken by patients (MHRA, 2004). Many aspects of its work have long come under repeated criticisms from patient groups, academics and social reformers (Medawar and Hardon, 2004). Critics think that the MHRA is biased in favour of pharmaceutical companies; allows biased research and the biased reporting of findings; and includes on its committees doctors who have benefited from drug companies' funding for their research or institutions (Medawar and Hardon, 2004). Until 2004, the MHRA refused to accept or pay attention to reports of adverse drug reactions from patients. Any reports that patients sent in were put to one side and disregarded, that is, discarded (member of MHRA staff, personal communication, 2004).

Deficiencies in the regulation of medicines have been compounded by some doctors' lack of attention to possible side effects when prescribing for patients. They have also been compounded by doctors choosing to select what information to provide to patients, rather than offering full information (Grime et al, 2007). Some professionals think that full information might deter patients from taking the medication (Grime et al, 2007). (This is deliberate covert coercion, Chapter Two.)

Millie Kieve set up APRIL in 1998, two years after her daughter, Karen, had fallen to her death from a window, probably as a psychiatric side effect (perhaps anxiety or confusion) of the medicines she had been prescribed for physical problems (Kieve, 2006). Her daughter had been given no warning and no information about possible psychiatric side effects when the medicines were prescribed. But Kieve found several papers and journals in the British Library that referred to the psychiatric adverse side effects of those medicines. So the side effects were known already. 'I felt I had opened a can of worms and that it was my destiny to do something about that wall of silence' (Kieve, 2004, p 4).

After her daughter's death in 1996, Kieve wrote to the Committee on Safety of Medicines (the relevant committee of the MHRA) giving details of the adverse effects of the medicines and anaesthetics that Karen had been given. They rejected her information. She decided that, if they would not listen to patients, she would. She set up APRIL and continues to collect and publicise information about the adverse side effects of various medicines. She also supports people who have been bereaved by medicine-induced deaths or who have suffered from medicine-induced distress or mental illness (Millie Kieve, personal communication, August 2008).

APRIL has campaigned about a variety of medicines whose adverse effects have been reported to it. It succeeded, for example, in getting the MHRA to review Dianette, a contraceptive pill that caused depression, and to change its labelling. It succeeded in persuading the General Medical Council (GMC) to include in its guidelines on medical education the need to educate medical students about adverse drug reactions. It puts on the only conferences about adverse drug reactions that are open to professionals and the public and that are not funded by pharmaceutical companies (Millie Kieve, personal communication, 2008).

APRIL's objective is to raise public and medical awareness of the psychiatric side effects of drugs for physical and psychiatric illnesses, and to so protect patients from them. It continues to urge the MHRA to review suspect medicines; and to require warnings on labels (Kieve, 2006).

APRIL has 6–8 trustees but no members (Millie Kieve, personal communication, 2008). The internet takes the place, in some ways, of the information-gathering, communication, publicity and support that members give each other in other patient groups. Radical activists dealing with straightforward, single issues will probably increasingly work in this way.

Forming a patient group is one way of seeking to change practices and standards. Some patients go on to develop wider expertise and can speak for the interests of patients in general (Chapter Seven). They are independent patient activists.

Independent activists

Independent activists often belong to several patient groups but also act in their own right, sitting on official committees, speaking at conferences and writing, not as representatives of any specific patient group. They generally build up portfolios of work, some paid (fees or honoraria), some unpaid. Their radicalisation shows the same pattern as that of activists who found patient groups. Like activists in recognised emancipation movements, they are admired by some dominant interest holders, feared by others. Those hostile to them often call them 'the usual suspects' (Hogg, 2009; and Chapter Nine).

Jean Robinson

An activist from conviction.

Jean Robinson had been a member of several patient groups when she became the chair of the Patients Association in 1973. The Patients Association was receiving up to 100 complaints a week. 'All of us who did the work [of helping the complainants] were radicalised by it. What impressed me was not just the extent of medical disasters, but also the profound additional damage inflicted when patients and the bereaved failed to get answers and were met with a stone wall of silence or outright lies' (Robinson, 1999, p 246).

Jean Robinson was appointed a lay member of the General Medical Council in 1979. She 'was an important and courageous critic within the Council ... [when she] confronted the Council with the inadequacy of its policies on poor clinical practice when seen from the viewpoint of the public rather than the medical profession', wrote Sir Donald Irvine, its president (Irvine, 2003, p 72). In 1988 she published a 'devastating critique of the Council's performance', *A patient voice at the GMC: A lay member's view of the General Medical Council* (Robinson, 1988; Irvine, 2003, p 72). She co-founded CERES, Consumers for Ethics in Research, a radical group concerned about medical research, in 1984; became the honorary research officer of AIMS; a committee member of POPAN, the Prevention of Professional Abuse Network, an organisation that helps people who have been emotionally abused by health or social care professionals, and aims to prevent further abuse; and a committee member of Action for Victims of Medical Accidents (AVMA) (Robinson, 1996a).

Mitzi Blennerhassett

An activist from personal experience.

While being treated for cancer of the anal canal, Mitzi Blennerhassett experienced a range of harms that left her badly shaken (Blennerhassett, 2008). When her consent for brachytherapy, a procedure in which implants (previously inserted under general anaesthesia) in the anal canal are connected by wires to a source of radioactivity, was sought, she was not told that the doctor who would insert the wires into the implants had never done it before and would be unsupervised. Moreover, while the doctor carried out the connecting procedure, he ignored her requests for pain relief (Blennerhassett, 1998). The long-term side effects of high-dose radiotherapy were not mentioned, nor the fact that the treatment proposed was a pioneering one, that is, an experimental or little-tried one. Her questions about her tumour's TNM (tumour, nodes, metastases) staging, which indicates prognosis, were evaded. She felt 'continually humiliated, manipulated, out of control' (Blennerhassett, 1998, p 1890).

Afterwards, she helped to found a patient support group, later running it. Posters that she put up in her local hospital to inform patients about the group were torn down. She became 'a reluctant activist', starting an activist group, Cancer Action Now (personal communications, 2007, 2008). Like Jean Robinson, she was later appointed to various national and Department of Health committees and working parties.

These eight accounts of radicalisation show us that the three conditions necessary for radicalisation were met. The first two can be refined specifically for healthcare.

The three conditions revisited

The first condition: perceived harm

Here the harm was harm to the self-as-body. Physical harms described in the activists' accounts were the replacement of a long-known, well-tolerated drug by one with worse, sometimes fatal, side effects (IDDT); high-dose radiotherapy regimes leading to injuries and sometimes to death (RAGE); drug-induced psychiatric states leading to accident or suicide (APRIL); untreated severe pain (Blennerhassett). The harms occurred in the course of treatments that professionals regarded as acceptable or good at the time. They were not the results of accidents or of practices or standards that most professionals would have regarded as poor. No one can take into account knowledge that lies in the future. But to the extent that doctors disregarded knowledge that was available, they repressed patients' interests in their own safety, as well as depriving them of information and choice.

Psychological harms were less clear cut and more difficult to assess, but patients suffered avoidable severe stress. Severe stress, especially for children, should be avoided whenever possible (Gould, 1968). If it cannot be avoided, it should not be inflicted on patients without warning them about it and giving them the chance to reject the procedure or ask to have it modified (Blennerhassett, 2008). AIMS and NAWCH were concerned with the psychological and developmental welfare of babies and children. AIMS members believed that separating healthy newborn babies from their mothers and feeding them by rigid schedules could harm them physically, by impeding breast feeding, as well as developmentally, by potentially impairing the relationship between them and their mothers. NAWCH members were mostly concerned about psychological stress or damage to children, but were alert to any evidence of physical harm. The distress of mothers forced to endure brutal regimes in maternity units and the anguish of parents forced to abandon their children crying in paediatric wards could seem almost unendurable to those experiencing them. Women in the Bristol trial felt that the remission of their cancer had been put at risk by the shock and distress of seeing, without any warning, the ominous findings from the trial that they believed was still going on (Goodare, 1996a).

The second condition: perception of personal indignity or injustice

Activists' accounts suggest that, in healthcare, the personal indignity or injustice can be seen as threats to the self-as-moral-agent. This concept is difficult to define and perhaps can be thought of as covering a cluster of feelings, differently expressed by different people. Patients have repeatedly said, from at least the 1960s, that they want "to be treated as a person", "not as a child", "not as stupid" (Chapters 1 and 7). Patients say this, even when they are satisfied with the treatment they have received. The sociologist Irving Zola said that patients did not want to be invalidated as persons (Zola, 1991). Another sociologist, Joanne Coyle, thought that threats to patients' personal or moral identity often seemed to underlie their accounts of their negative experiences in healthcare (Coyle, 1999). She based this conclusion on interviews with a sub sample of 21 women and 20 men, from a sample of 1,640 people in a household survey in London, who had said they had experienced problems with their healthcare (Coyle, 1999). The 41 patients' problems included misdiagnoses and inadequate investigations, and some had felt 'dehumanised, objectified, stereotyped, disempowered and devalued' (Coyle, 1999, p 724). In criticising their healthcare, respondents 'cast aspersions' on the professional integrity of the doctors and nurses who had treated them, while preserving 'their own moral identity by demonstrating competence, knowledge, rationality, reasonableness and concern for others' (Coyle, 1999, p 723).

The concept of moral agency seems to fit these descriptions. The self-as-moral-agent tries to take right action, to act in accord with its responsibilities to itself, its family and its wider community (Chapter Six). The self-as-moral-agent is closely related to autonomy, because when professionals respect patients' autonomy, patients are free to take the actions they think right, without coercion. Being treated with indignity or injustice affronts that sense of self-as-moral-agent.

Patients' moral agency can be threatened or affronted in many ways. Some routine practices, like booking several patients for the same time to see the same doctor in out-patients departments, can surprise and offend patients, because they breach ordinary social norms of courtesy. They are probably seldom threatening enough to radicalise anyone, but they may pave the way for later radicalisation. Other policies and practices may have elements of coercion that can contribute to radicalisation. They can be divided into overtly coercive ways and covertly coercive ways, depending upon how clear the threats are to the patients threatened (Chapter Two).

Overt coercion

The purpose of overt coercion is to control patients' or relatives' actions. So policies and practices that are overtly coercive have to be made known to those who are expected to comply with them. Patients may accept them. Or they may become aware that they are prevented from acting as they think and feel right, either by being restricted from doing something or by being forced to do it. They may define that experience as oppression. So it is unsurprising that radical patient activism often began as opposition to overtly coercive policies and practices. Examples are NAWCH and AIMS.

Health professionals' and institutions' resistances to requests to change coercive policies can radicalise activists further. Refusals and resistances can harden activists' determination by calling on their pride, skill and courage. Resistances can also prompt activists to scrutinise other policies and practices: to uproot them and shake the earth off them to examine their effects on patients' experiences or on their interests.

Covert coercion

The effect of covert coercion, like that of overt coercion, is to control patients' actions. But covert coercion is more complex. Professionals or managers may think that covert coercion is a legitimate form of social control, because the boundary between legitimate and illegitimate control can be problematic or disputed (Kemper, 2001). Or professionals and managers may be so accustomed to what they do that they do not see it as either coercion or control: it is just the way things are. Dominant interest holders accept the status quo that supports their interests, partly by seeing it as natural. But patients may experience the status quo as a threat to their autonomy or their moral agency, if they 'awaken' to it, that is, if it becomes visible to them or if they see it as no longer natural and legitimate. Then they may experience it as oppression (Chapter Two).

When patients complain about not being listened to, being misled or inadequately informed, commentators often put it down to professionals' lack of communication or interpersonal skills (Tattersall and Ellis, 1998). This may, or may not, be a factor. But here we are looking at the effects on patients, not at professionals' reasons or circumstances. The accounts show that patients' sense of moral agency can be affronted because the validity of what they say is denied or they are misled in some way or treated without respect.

Denial of validity

1. Disbelieving what patients say. The founders of IDDT were not believed when they said that synthetic insulin was worse for them, and for many other patients, than animal insulin. 'Not listening to patients – is it instinctive?' was the title of an editorial by Jenny Hirst in the IDDT *April 2005 Newsletter* (Hirst, 2005a).

2. Disregarding what they say or request. Doctors treating Blennerhassett paid no attention to her protests about the pain she was feeling. They did not explain why they could not use a painkiller. Indeed,

there was no reason; and that hospital now offers patients analgesia (Blennerhassett, 2008).

3. Not answering their questions. Blennerhassett found this with her questions about the staging and the possible recurrence of her cancer.

4. Paying no or scant attention to reports, criticisms (constructive or otherwise) or suggestions that patients or their relatives make after the episode of treatment is over. Patients' hope that their experiences and suggestions could help doctors and managers provide better care for future patients are nullified when this happens. IDDT and APRIL exemplify this.

Patients' surprise, anger, disappointment or despair when what they said was disregarded is a mark of how deeply they felt that their moral agency was discounted.

Misleading patients

1. Lying in answer to questions. Goodare's oncologist said that tamoxifen had no side effects. A truthful answer would have been "we don't yet know what all the possible side effects of tamoxifen might be, but as an anti-oestrogen we might expect it to have some".

2. Withholding information about the possible adverse reactions or complications of the treatments offered or prescribed. RAGE, APRIL, IDDT and Blennerhassett exemplify this. This withholding is akin to the withholding of information about post-mortems from parents at Alder Hey and Bristol (Chapter Two). It is strongly coercive.

3. Failing to be open about the status or experience of the health professional carrying out the procedure or treatment. Blennerhassett's experience with a doctor carrying out a procedure for the first time, and unsupervised, was an example.

These three points are relevant to patients' consent to procedures and treatments. All medical interventions carry risks of possible harmful effects as well as hoped-for benefits (Smith and Adams, 2003). Patients, either alone or with their doctors, have to weigh the kinds of possible harms and how likely they are to occur against the value to them of the hoped-for goods or benefits. Any withholding of accurate information or of uncertainty about what the risks might be negates the protection afforded to patients by the ethical requirement to obtain their consent to treatment (General Medical Council, 1998). Patients must be able, if they so wish, to decide whether to accept a proposed treatment, accepting its risks, or to reject it or to seek another opinion. Preventing them from doing that is an affront to them as moral agents. Withholding information is coercive if it encourages patients to consent to what they would have refused, if they had known, or if it prevents them from asking for something they were not told about (Chapter Two).

◊◊ "If only they had told me…": Margaret King (Chapter Five), reflecting on her experience of radiotherapy and its aftermath (personal communication, 1997). ◊◊

4. Patients can also be misled when professionals or managers fail to acknowledge to the patient that the kind of harm done to him or her was, or could have been, already known about. RAGE members were especially enraged when the radiologist or clinician to whom they showed their damaged bodies asserted that their case was unique. The founder of APRIL felt there was 'a wall of silence', something that had been built on purpose, around the adverse psychiatric effects of some medicines.

This is linked to not paying attention to what patients say or not regarding what they report as valid. Stories, anecdotes and data offered by patients that could have been recorded and collated are disregarded (APRIL).

Lack of respect

Failing to apologise to patients, even after admitting publicly that what was done was erroneous or defective, is a breach of 'ordinary' social norms. BSSG members felt that they should have been apologised to for their distressing experiences of reading that their lives had been shortened while, as far as they knew, the research was still in progress.

◊◊ 'I remember where I was when I heard I had doubled my chances of dying of breast cancer by going to the Bristol Cancer Help Centre … Never at any time was I approached to discuss my misgivings, and like the other women used for the research I have not received an adequate apology for my wasted time and effort and distress,' wrote Sheila Hancock, the distinguished actress (Hancock, 1996, p ix). ◊◊

Evident harm alerts patients to situations, issues and standards that they might not have thought about at all, had the harm not occurred. A successful treatment, during or after which no adverse reactions or complications occur, may make patients forgive, or even not notice, that information was deficient, that risks were inadequately explained or other possible treatments were not mentioned. Health professionals' view that only patients who have met with some unusual mishap become activists has some truth in it, inasmuch as personal experience of harm to the self-as-body and threats to the self-as-moral-agent can be so cogent a motive for taking social action. But 'unusual' is relative; and what is unusual can be at least as important as something that is usual. When patients complain, they are more forgiving if what they say is believed and if they receive an explanation of what went wrong and a promise to prevent the same thing happening again, as well as an apology, than if they do not (Lloyd-Bostock, 1999). Harm seems to be more easily borne when the moral agency of the patient has not been affronted.

The third condition: a sense of social efficacy

Efficacy is the capacity to produce effects (Little et al, 1936). A sense of efficacy is the confidence that one can cause changes to be made. It probably starts from a sense of personal efficacy, an ability to get things done. A sense of social efficacy is a belief that other people have had similar experiences, will want to join in working for change, and that acting collectively can bring about change (Mansbridge, 2001a). In healthcare, this social aspect marks the difference between patient activism and patients' private dissatisfactions, informal and formal complaints and recourses to the law.

Once a radical patient group gets going, its members can begin to define their values, perceptions and definitions collectively. They can begin to create the group's own knowledge and ethical bases (Chapter Five). Its members can support and reinforce each other in the skills and in the courage that is needed to take action against the status quo. Founding or joining a group of like-minded people is often the first step in bringing about social and political change (Chapters 1 and 3). Groups also are seen as socially legitimate; and that is important for patients whose words are so easily ignored (Zola, 1991).

All the accounts of activists' actions show their sense of personal and social efficacy.

'Something should be done', then doing it (AIMS); 'I felt ... that it was my destiny to do something ...', then doing it (APRIL).

Comparing radicalisation with the birth of 'oppositional consciousness' in recognised emancipation movements

These activists' accounts let us compare the three general conditions that social scientists postulate are necessary for the development of what they call 'oppositional consciousness' or 'awakening to political consciousness' with the specific ones that seem to apply to radicalisation in healthcare.

1. *Members of an oppressed group are prompted to act by the personal indignities and harms suffered because they are members of the oppressed group, that is, a subordinate group subject to the unjust use of power by the dominant group (Mansbridge, 2001a).*

   The coercions that we see in the activists' accounts are instances of the unjust use of power by a dominant group or groups. The coercions were personal, in the behaviours of professionals towards individual patients; collective, in the policies and customary practices of groups of professionals; and social, in the assumptions and actions explicitly or implicitly agreed between professionals and healthcare and other social institutions like pharmaceutical companies and the agencies that regulate medicines, like the MHRA.

2. *A sense of identity with other people in the same situation (the oppressed group) is necessary for radicalisation (Goodwin et al, 2001; Mansbridge and Morris, 2001; Klandermans, 1997).*

   There are always more people who are non-activists than activists, even though both may seem to be in the same situation or suffering the same plight (Kemper, 2001; Chapter Nine). About 7% of the original 334 women in the Bristol arm of the trial joined BSSG. (The group's founders had to try to reach the women through patient groups' networks because they did not have access to the researchers' mailing list, and so did not know how many women knew about the group (Goodare, 1996a).) For AIMS, NAWCH, RAGE and IDDT, people in the same situation and ready to join a group were found through newspaper or other publicity. For APRIL, people were ready to send anecdotes and opinion to Kieve through the internet.

   Although the memberships of the groups varied over time, only a few activists were needed to form a group to take social action, then sustain it for many years or until the desired changes to policy or practice took place.

3. *A sense of efficacy or 'agency' is a necessary condition for the development of oppositional consciousness (Mansbridge, 2001b; Klandermans, 1997).*

All the accounts here show a sense of efficacy, some explicitly.

In addition to meeting these three major conditions, the accounts show that the patients who were radicalised experienced the emotions common to people 'awakened' in recognised emancipation movements.

4. *When 'awakening' takes place in recognised emancipation movements, unquestioning or unconscious subscription to dominant interests, perceptions and values is lost for ever.*

New beliefs and ways of looking at familiar things take their place (Mansbridge, 2001a). From disillusion comes illumination. This has been compared with crossing the boundary into another country, a country from which one can never go back (Cross, 1995).

For 'awakening' in healthcare, the loss of the belief that doctors and other health professionals always act in the interests of patients, whether individual patients or patients collectively, seems to be crucial. The loss was expressed through activists' sense of surprise, shock and disappointment. It contradicted the socially accepted professional ideology that supported dominant interests. In its place, activists began to identify and define patients' interests, as patients identified them, or would identify them, if they knew they were threatened, and to judge whether they conflicted with or were compatible with professionals' interests (Chapter One). These processes both create and reflect new knowledge (Chapter Five).

5. *Anger towards the dominant group fuels activists' actions against it (Mansbridge, 2001b; Polletta and Amenta, 2001).*

Anger is explicit in some activists' accounts. But a single word does not cover all the feelings of dismay, disillusion, despair and anguish that some activists felt as they became radicalised.

6. *The strong feelings of anger and injustice can be channelled into positive action (Mansbridge, 2001a).*

Strong feelings can be the basis for protest, for political challenge and for strategic thought (Goodwin et al, 2001a). Strong feelings are needed to oppose dominant interests, with their pervasive institutional and structural support. Much political effort is needed (Alford, 1975).

The activist groups here acted politically and thought strategically in defining their goals and planning what actions to take.

◊◊ '… it was only through becoming involved in the campaign for our rights as patients that I was able to work through my feelings of outrage,' wrote a member of BSSG (Charles, 1996, p 39). ◊◊

◊◊ 'You've got to feel huge passion and indignation, and that's got to be the unifying thing,' said Jan Millington of RAGE (Hanley and Staley, 2006, p 96). ◊◊

7. *Strong feelings and convictions support a sense of 'principled commitment' (Mansbridge, 2001b).*

Some of the activists in this chapter have worked as activists, most of the time unpaid, for more than 40 years.

Conclusion

Radicalisation usually starts from personal experience. But reading or hearing about patients' experiences can radicalise (Robinson, 1999). Radicalisation can take place through identification with, or a sense of connectedness to, those who have suffered or may suffer from some specific harm (Williamson, 1992). Intense intellectual, emotional or moral convictions often come in, as they do in those who work, for example, to free domestic or wild animals from human cruelty. But personal experience, direct or vicarious, lies at the roots of radical activism in healthcare. Members' personal experience of being oppressed makes emancipation movements different from other social movements (Mansbridge, 2001a; Chapter Three).

The conditions that led to the radicalisation of the patient activists described here are like those that lead to awakening or the development of oppositional consciousness in recognised emancipation movements.

FIVE

Radical activists' new knowledge

*... [activist groups'] efforts to construct a new kind of science –
one which uses a combination of observation, anecdote, dialogue,
complaints and human input as well as the available scientific,
sociological and psychological evidence – to reach its conclusions
regarding appropriate care, and to identify problems and
opportunities for change.*

(Pat Thomas, AIMS member, 2002, p 6)

Introduction

Activists' decision that something needs to be done to oppose low
standards of care or oppressive practices and to propose higher standards
instead means that they have to assemble evidence and argument to
make their case. They have to draw on the knowledge they have built
up, their new knowledge. This chapter analyses what new knowledge
consists of, and gives two detailed examples of new knowledge and of
how activists use it.

Patient groups' knowledge

All social groups build up a knowledge base unique to their group,
drawn from their experiences, perceptions and insights (Baggott et al,
2005). Radical groups and individuals search for additional knowledge,
taking it eclectically from various academic disciplines (Fletcher, 2002).
If they cannot find the evidence they need in one discipline, they
look in another (Williamson, 1992). They cross academic boundaries,
blend different kinds and levels of knowledge and draw out new
ideas, to create their new, emergent or activist expert knowledge.
Activists use their new knowledge for thinking, but also for action.
It enables them to judge proposals, policies, practices and standards as
being in patients' interests or as undermining them. It is part of their
armoury of opposition or counter-expertise (Hess, 2004; Williamson,
2008a). Radical patient activists construct their new knowledge from
their perspective of alignment with patients. Their new knowledge
reinforces their beliefs and drives their actions; and their passion can
give intellectual and political force to what they say (Chapter Four).

Activists' new knowledge

Activists' new knowledge is a network of clusters of knowledge and ideas that each group creates from various fields of knowledge and thought. All radical patient groups probably hold some ideas in common, including the values and principles that guide their actions (Chapter Six). But each group specialises. Activist patient groups and individual activists need not and cannot master the whole of any medical, scientific or social scientific discipline. (Professionals and academics may feel puzzled or resentful about this. "How can they know anything about what it has taken me 25 years to learn?") Activist members of patient groups build up their specialised knowledge within the group and during their work for it. Independent activists coming to a clinical specialty new to them have to learn quickly about the practices, standards and issues in that specialty before they can bring their perspectives to bear upon them.

◊◊ "It's a steep learning curve." (independent patient activist, on moving from maternity care to anaesthesia, personal communication, 2002) ◊◊

What is new knowledge about? It is about the effects of professionals' and corporate rationalisers' actions or inactions upon patients. Linking patients' experiences and judgements with healthcare professionals' actions, and drawing conclusions from this linkage, constitutes activists' new knowledge or 'new kind of science'. It combines experiential and scientific knowledge (Thomas, P., 2002; Martin, 2008) It often starts from the problems, dissatisfactions and harms that patients experience (Chapter Four). As activists build up their new knowledge, it comes to include their definitions of what are good and desirable standards of treatment and care and of ethics. At the roots of activists' new knowledge lie concerns about what patients tell them.

Starting from what patients tell them about the harmful, or more rarely, the good, healthcare that they have experienced, activists study what is known about the relevant professional practice, assumptions, arguments and research evidences on which it is based. Doctors' clinical knowledge has a higher social status than patients' experiential knowledge. But in patient groups, patients critical of clinicians' knowledge that has not served them well tend to attribute greater value to patients' experiential knowledge than to that clinical knowledge (Whelan, 2007). Members of a group may use their experiential knowledge to discredit clinicians' and medical researchers' claims to reliable knowledge (Whelan, 2007).

They also consider clinicians' experiential knowledge as less reliable than evidence from medical research (Whelan, 2007). Clinicians' experiential and anecdotal knowledge, however, like patients' anecdotal knowledge, can open up new ideas or issues. Constructing 'a new kind of science' requires challenging the statuses of different kinds of knowledge drawn from disparate fields.

In political terms, new knowledge is about the effects of dominant interests or dominant interest holders on repressed interests or repressed interest holders. New knowledge tends to act against the status quo and is like the 'consciousness raising' of recognised emancipation movements: it uncovers hidden harms. IDDT's uncovering of the adverse side effects of synthetic insulin, with which doctors and pharmaceutical companies were about to replace animal insulin, is an example (Chapter Four). Sometimes the harms are already known but not acted on; then activists' public exposure of them, as with RAGE and radiotherapy (Chapter Four), constitutes consciousness raising. These uncoverings and exposures are the first step in lifting repression from patients' interests.

New knowledge can be called new for several reasons.

New knowledge is recent

It is recent, dating from the late 1950s and early 1960s, when patients began to take action, forming patient groups, sharpening their perspectives and building up their knowledge bases.

Unlike professional knoweldge, new knowledge focuses on harms

New knowledge is new because it focuses on harms. Medical knowledge, by contrast, focuses mainly on the good that medicine does. Medical teaching is mainly about what medicine can do to alleviate pain, sickness and distress: it is about making patients better. Doctors resist the idea that their actions can harm patients, partly because, like the rest of us, their self-esteem depends upon their belief that the actions they take are right (Chapter Nine). Also, the uncertainties of medical knowledge and the vagaries of the body's responses to clinical interventions can obscure iatrogenic (doctor-induced) harms. Doctors' ideological belief that they act in patients' interests, and political and social structures that help to sustain that belief, can blind doctors to those harms. So can the repression of patients' interests (Chapter Two). Doctors' inattention to the side effects of drugs, and their perfunctoriness in reporting them to the regulatory authority, illustrate this enduring problem (Medawar and Hardon, 2004; Chapter Four, APRIL (p 55); Chapter Seven). So do dramatic disasters.

◊◊ Thousands of patients with haemophilia in the US and Europe were infected by HIV (the human immunodeficiency virus) in products made from blood because haematologists and regulatory agencies failed to act quickly to stop the distribution of the clotting factor, factor VIII, after the blood used to make it had been contaminated by HIV (Resnik, 1999). That failure resulted in the deaths from AIDS (acquired immunodeficiency syndrome) of many patients with haemophilia, and left the prospect of living with HIV for many others (Resnik, 1999). Doctors' denial, paternalism and hubris (excessive self-confidence) contributed to the disaster in some countries (Resnik, 1999). ◊◊

Doctors and corporate rationalisers tend to shy away from doing or commissioning research that could look for or at harms.

◊◊ Some doctors have seen 'nothing wrong in setting out deliberately to prove that patients like the care being provided' by using biased questionnaires they have drawn up themselves (Robinson, 1996b, p 41). ◊◊

◊◊ Handbooks for patient involvement managers or health service staff seeking patients' views in focus groups, interviews or questionnaires sometimes advise staff to stay away from 'sensitive' topics and to avoid questioning patients about aspects of the service over which those staff have no control (York Health Services NHS Trust, 2001). This prevents patients from saying what they really think about their care. It also prevents patients' concerns from reaching managers higher up in the organisation, who could do something about them. ◊◊

◊◊ The Healthcare Commission, a national body for the audit and inspection of healthcare, in commissioning a national survey of women who had had babies in February 2007 excluded from the sample women whose babies had died perinatally or who were under 16 when their babies were born (Healthcare Commission, 2007). As two especially vulnerable groups of mothers, their experiences and judgements of those experiences would have been important, quite apart from the Commission's deliberate introduction of bias into the sample. ◊◊

These examples show how the repression of patients' interests can be sustained by omitting certain questions or excluding certain respondents. Omissions and exclusions may be due to researchers' political cautiousness or to their fear that a specific funding body will not pay for research that might produce disquieting findings. Or researchers may themselves be aligned with professionals or with corporate rationalisers. Few academic researchers in the UK have explored patients' views and feelings empathetically, perhaps because they might be criticised by other social scientists for being 'subjective' (Thomas, C., 2007).

Politically, healthcare professionals have not needed to inquire into patients' views; that is a privilege of dominance. Besides, disturbing the status quo by uncovering any unfortunate aspects of it would be disloyal to other dominant interest holders (Chapter Nine). At another level of explanation, psychoanalytic theory tells us that healthcare professionals have psychological, organisational and unconscious defences against examining too closely or feeling too acutely patients' plight or the possible harm that their own well-intended actions can do to patients (Menzies, 1959). Even when staff are aware of harmful practices, they may disavow that knowledge, deploring it but doing nothing about it (Menzies Lyth, 1988a). The experiences of doctors who become patients or of midwives who have babies can surprise and dismay them, however much they had thought they understood their patients' feelings.

◊◊ Until she had an aggressive cancer, Dr Jane Poulson, an academic physician who had practised palliative care medicine in a teaching hospital, had thought that she was a particularly empathetic doctor who heard her patients' stories (Poulson, 1998). She had noticed that few patients seemed encouraged to hear that there had been recent 'tremendous advances in technology and supportive care' for cancer (Poulson, 1998, p 1845). But she had not realised how emotionally and physically devastating some treatments for cancer could be; how postponements of investigations or delays in telling patients the results greatly increased their anxiety; or how shattering it was for them to be told they were not eligible for a study or clinical trial of an experimental treatment that might save their lives (Poulson, 1998). ◊◊

In contrast to professionals, patient activists want and need to keep in touch with patients' experiences, views and judgements, politically and pragmatically. It is part of their everyday work and a major source of their credibility and authority. Though they are distressed to see or to hear about poor care, it provides them with more evidence and argument, as well as reinforcing their commitment to their work.

New knowledge seeks to understand dominant interest holders and their interests

Although professionals need not seek nor study patients' experiences, views, values or motives, patient activists must try to understand those of professionals and corporate rationalisers. Repressed interest holders have to study dominant interest holders more carefully than vice versa (Alford, 1975; Williamson, 1992). This aspect makes their knowledge new in the sense of different from many professionals' lack of knowledge of repressed interest holders' interests, values and views (Chapter Two).

New knowledge is biased towards repressed interests

Medical science and research are biased towards dominant interests (Hogg, 1988). These accepted biases are part of the pervasive social structural support for dominant interests (Chapter Two). Radical patient activists' knowledge is biased towards repressed interests. This bias is new in healthcare.

The sources of new knowledge

Radical patient activism's new knowledge has six main sources: (1) lay knowledge; (2) lifeworld knowledge; (3) patients' and patient activists' experiences; (4) medicine and other natural sciences; (5) social sciences; and (6) other social movements. Individual activists and groups draw on different elements of these sources at different times in the development of their knowledge and expertise and in their strategic use of it. Thomas's word 'available' (in the quotation at the head of this chapter) reminds us that people cannot draw on data or theories that have not yet come into being. Patient activists in the 1960s and early 1970s, for example, could not have read Lukes's or Alford's key works on the nature and distribution of power, and dominance, first published in 1974 and 1975 (Lukes, 2005; Alford, 1975). Iris Marion Young's important book on social justice and oppression was not published until 1990 (Young, 1990).

1. Lay knowledge

Lay knowledge is the ordinary social, ethical and common-sense knowledge that 'ordinary' lay people or members of the public share. Every highly trained, highly specialised professional group loses some lay values and ethical norms, replacing them with others of their own that separate them from lay people, a separation that both serves the group instrumentally and may desensitise it emotionally (Bosk, 1979). The ethical element is especially important because medical ethics differs in some ways from lay ethics.

> ◊◊ The discovery that children's organs were retained post-mortem without their parents' knowledge or consent at Alder Hey Hospital in Liverpool and at the Royal Infirmary in Bristol breached lay ethics and public norms (Royal Liverpool Children's Inquiry, 2001; Bristol Royal Infirmary Inquiry, 2000). Some healthcare professionals think that the secret practice was not wrong in the past, merely judged so with hindsight (Underwood, 2003). They are mistaken. Revealing the secrecy of the practice years ago would almost certainly have elicited the same shocked reactions from the public. ◊◊

Some of what happens backstage, though not secret – things done out of patients' sight, or things done or left undone by tacit agreement among professionals – would also incur patients' and the public's disapproval (Williamson, 2000b). Disjunctions between professional and ordinary social norms and values come up when lay people work with professionals.

> ◊◊ "You are the conscience of the College," said the president of a medical royal college to the lay member on its Council (lay member, a patient activist, personal observation, 2000). ◊◊

Lay knowledge, however, can be strongly influenced by long-standing, perhaps outmoded, medical ideas. So, for example, lay people may assume that births in hospital must always be safer than births at home, though this is not so (Tew, 1990). Lay knowledge can also rely too heavily on common sense that supports dominant interests (Chapter Eight). But lay knowledge and values form the basis from which radical patient activism starts to build up its specialised knowledge. Activists' specialised knowledge remains more closely in touch with ordinary values and norms than professionals' specialised knowledge, partly because activists are in constant touch with patients who can speak freely to them as equals with shared experiences of patienthood.

2. Lifeworld knowledge

Lifeworld knowledge, in the context of healthcare, consists of lay people's everyday ideas and perspectives about illness, health and medical care (Williams and Popay, 2006). It comes from personal, family and traditional knowledge (Williams and Popay, 2006). Lifeworld knowledge, like lay knowledge, can be developed into specialised or expert knowledge that retains a lay perspective: people with lifeworld knowledge facing some possible threat to the environment or their health, from a river they fear may be polluted, for example, can extend that knowledge into expertise (Williams and Popay, 2006). They extend it for the same reason that patient activists do: expertise is usually needed to challenge or oppose dominant interest holders effectively.

Lifeworld knowledge is not sharply separate from ordinary lay knowledge. Lifeworld perspectives are probably carried into patient activists' creation of new knowledge by, for example, predisposing them to be sceptical about the safety of medicines. Some activists value simple traditional remedies and complementary therapies; they seldom view them with the disdain that some healthcare professionals feel. A lifeworld tradition of home births passes down from mother to daughter to granddaughter in some families (Nadine Edwards, personal communication, 2007).

3. Patients' and patient activists' experiential knowledge

Activists' own experiences as patients may prompt them to become activists (Chapter Four). Or what a patient group does 'may strike a chord' with someone unaffected by direct experience, who then joins the group. But activists' experience as activists rather than as patients is probably their most important source of new knowledge.

Patients often get in touch with patient groups who they think will be sympathetic to their concerns; patients' oral and written accounts of their experiences of episodes of healthcare are a unique resource for patient groups. The accounts show what current healthcare is like. Sometimes they uncover new problems or provide new ideas or insights. Patients' accounts are subjective; that is their value. Their descriptions of what has happened are often objective in the sense of accurate, though, like most descriptions, they may be incomplete. Patients may misinterpret or misjudge some of what they observe, or, indeed, cannot observe, if it takes place out of their sight. But the accounts' combinations of objective description and subjective feeling and interpretation provide rich material for analysis and synthesis.

◊◊ Jean Robinson described AIMS' way of using anecdotal evidence from patients and their relatives: 'We watch, wait, see if it's a blip, network with other groups to see if they are getting the same thing, and look into the literature and statistics. And … we often bounce our findings off academics in the field, talk to practitioners and pass the information round the AIMS committee.… We use anecdotal evidence only when we have a substantial quantity, when we are sure of the quality and when we have put it into context' (Robinson, 2004/5, p 15). ◊◊

Activists' appointments to other bodies, like health service governance bodies, regulatory bodies, research ethics committees, working or liaison groups, provide another field for their observations and collections of evidence. Some moderately radical activists set up as independent researchers or healthcare consultants. (A very radical activist would probably have few customers.) So activists can draw on diverse experiences and insights in their construction of new knowledge.

Activists' accounts of their experiences and conclusions can be highly influential. Jean Robinson's insider's account of the way the General Medical Council worked, *A patient voice at the GMC: A lay member's view of the General Medical Council*, published in 1988 (Chapter Four), helped to bring about the reforms made to the GMC in the 1990s (Robinson, 1988; Irvine, 2003).

4. Medicine and other natural or physical sciences

Medicine, and its clinical knowledge and practice, are crucial to patient activism. Though activists are unlikely to discover something entirely new clinically or scientifically, they can pick up trends in patients' experiences, problems and disbenefits much earlier than doctors seem able or inclined to do (Pat Thomas, 2002). This is partly because patients tell patient groups about their experiences, whereas a clinician may see few or no patients who have been harmed. It is partly because activists' study of research literature alerts them to the kinds of problems to expect. But information about patients' negative experiences, feelings and views is unlikely to be welcome to, or even believed by, all doctors, though radical doctors may welcome hearing about what patients perceive as poor practice (Chapter Nine). Doctors sometimes seem reluctant or unable to believe that patients experience problems or harms until those harms are officially recognised and recorded by their own professional bodies (Robinson, 1993). So one of activists' tasks is to approach professional, governmental or other official bodies, in person or by sending written comments, with details about problems and with proposals about policies, practices and standards that could reduce or prevent them (Chapter Four).

Radical patient activists who address clinical matters must learn the relevant medical terminology. Using clinicians' vocabulary and knowing about the technical aspects of their work is usually necessary for arguing a case for change in practices or standards (Arksey, 1994; Batt, 1994; Oliver et al, 2001). Activists may argue for new ways of doing things, new standards. Or they may remind professionals of the high ethical and clinical standards they profess. Dominant interest holders have to be challenged on their own ground; that is a privilege of dominance. If the people who talk with them do not speak their language, they allow dominance to flourish.

◊◊ "Knowing the other side's literature is what counts; then you can criticise it effectively." (Radical activist, personal communication, 2008) ◊◊

Talking to doctors in their own language earns their respect, inclines them to pay attention to what is said and makes it more likely that they will understand it.

◊◊ In a discussion group with anaesthetists at a conference in 2002, I noticed that one consultant anaesthetist made no pretence of listening to me. When he began to speak of the importance of emphasising the safety of anaesthesia, I, provoked, said, "If you think that anaesthesia is safe, you haven't read the latest CEPOD [Confidential Enquiry into Perioperative Deaths] Report." His attitude changed instantly: he became polite, almost deferential, and later offered to fetch me a cup of tea. ◊◊

Some lay people's often-expressed hope that doctors will use only simplified or lay terms in talking with lay people and patients can be an inadvertent way of repressing patients' interests. It deprives patients of the technical terms they need when talking with other patients or with doctors. It hampers patients' attempts to look for further information independently. It anchors patients in their low status. But ways to enhance clinicians' and patients' shared understanding of terms in clinical consultations need to be found (Koch-Weser et al, 2009).

Another common fallacy is that, if activists become familiar with professionals and professional knowledge, they will adopt professional perceptions and values – will 'go native'. Alford noted that dominant interest holders cooptated patient activists as a way of repressing patients' interests (Alford, 1975). Cooptation, inviting people to be members of a prestigious group in order to win them over to its views, is always a danger when weaker interest holders mingle with more powerful ones. But the danger is less for radical patient activists than for conservative patient activists, whose interests are already aligned with professionals' interests (Chapters 3 and 8). For radical activists, the reverse of winning over is more likely. The more that radical patient activists know about professional assumptions and practices, the more they see to deplore in the profession collectively, as well as to admire in many individual professionals (Robinson, 1988). Activists can detach the personal from the political: married feminists can love their husbands, patient activists in professional–patient activist working groups can like their medical colleagues.

5. Social sciences

The social sciences are important sources of new knowledge. Their various disciplines offer different kinds and levels of ways of looking at things. They can be drawn on for explanations of what can be observed in healthcare, professionals' and corporate rationalisers' behaviour, and power relationships (Chapter Two). In addition, social scientists' detailed studies of specific situations can provide evidence that can be used in arguing for change.

Just as activists' approach to medical science is selective, so it is to social science. They take ideas and evidence from its disciplines eclectically, without respecting disciplinary boundaries (Fletcher, 2002). This approach may puzzle or offend some social scientists, just as encroaching on medical knowledge may surprise or antagonise some doctors. To social scientists, activists' new knowledge can seem 'a muddle of perspectives' with a weak evidence base rather than proper knowledge (Fletcher, 2002, p 91). This may also be partly because new knowledge is still being created, because it can be threatening, and because it is hard to capture and codify.

6. Other social movements

Early AIMS, National Childbirth Trust (NCT) and NAWCH members knew that they were influenced by the women's movement (Patricia Wilkie, early NCT member, personal communication, 2006). Some activists looked to other emancipatory movements in the US for inspiration (Chapter Six).

Two examples of the sources and uses of new knowledge

Patient activists draw on and combine these six sources of new knowledge, according to their purposes. Here are two detailed examples of how they do this. The first is about activists' use of social science knowledge in the creation of new knowledge, the second is about medical and scientific knowledge. Both examples show how activist patient groups gathered data about the extent of the harms to patients; put together knowledge from various sources; and proposed remedies in patient care or in research to higher standards. Both groups engaged with radical and conservative professionals and with corporate rationalisers. One group, NAWCH, has succeeded in its primary objective; the other, RAGE, not yet. Chapter Four gave brief accounts of these two radical patient groups. Founded 30 years apart, they had different objectives; but they met the same difficulties.

Knowledge from social science knowledge – NAWCH – founded 1961

NAWCH, the National Association for the Welfare of Children in Hospital, is a patient group that from its beginning drew on social sciences to argue its case against some accepted practices and standards. It did not concern itself directly with clinical treatments, though it challenged matters that doctors and nurses deemed clinical, matters to do with how they worked and with how treatments were given.

At the beginning of the 20th century, children in hospital were seldom allowed to be visited by their parents, sometimes for months on end (Hales-Tooke, 1973). In the 1940s, after the Second World War, psychoanalytically trained people in London, some who had been refugees from continental Europe, like Anna Freud, began to look at the effects on children of separation from their parents. They studied children evacuated from cities during the war, children in nurseries, in orphanages and in long-stay hospitals (Robertson, 1958; Cohen,

1964). Work at the Tavistock Institute of Human Relations by Dr John Bowlby, a medically qualified psychoanalyst, and James Robertson, a psychiatric social worker and psychoanalyst, concluded that young children need a stable and responsive mother-figure for their healthy emotional and intellectual development. Young children should not be separated from their mothers, especially not in times of stress, such as a stay in hospital (Robertson, 1958). In 1952 Robertson made a film, *A two-year-old goes to hospital*, to try to bring home to health professionals how much distress and disturbance young children could suffer from separation (Robertson, 1953). The film evoked much hostility towards Robertson from doctors and nurses (Cohen, 1964).

◊◊ Robertson's campaign was probably partly prompted by personal experience: his own daughter had been rushed into hospital in 1945: '... we weren't allowed to visit for ten days. Our daughter was transformed from a confident toddler to a very insecure little person, a condition lasting for years' (Cohen, 1964, p 63). ◊◊

In 1956 the Ministry of Health commissioned a study of the arrangements for the welfare of children in hospital, excluding clinical care (Hales-Tooke, 1973). (The exclusion of clinical care from the study was a mark of clinicians' dominance.) Published in 1959 as the Platt Report, it recommended that visiting to children be unrestricted; that mothers be admitted to hospital with their children; and that the training of doctors and nurses give them greater understanding of children's and families' emotional and social needs (Hales-Tooke, 1973). The Ministry of Health adopted the report as policy and asked all hospitals to implement its recommendations. They did not.

In 1961, Robertson's film was shown on television and led to the founding of NAWCH (Chapter Four). After seeing his film, the founding members of NAWCH went to see James Robertson. He advised them to read up the subject (mother–child bonding, the Platt Report, and so on) before they started visiting hospitals or met government officials or ministers (Peg Belson, personal communication, 2008). Later, national NAWCH regularly sent reading lists and photocopies of papers and articles to local NAWCH groups. They included 'The Story of Dawn' (Chapter Four) and a study describing how, in spite of the benefits to children of admitting their mothers with them, nurses in Rubery Hill Hospital in Birmingham preferred to have children admitted on their own; they were easier to nurse and more rewarding emotionally (Brain and Maclay, 1968). These papers helped to shape and spread NAWCH's radical culture.

Some NAWCH members also read psychoanalytically-based paperback books addressed to the general public, like James Robertson's *Young children in hospital*, 1958; D. W. Winnicott's *The child, the family, and the outside world*, 1964; John Bowlby's *Child care and the growth of love*, 1965. Isabel Menzies' paper 'The functioning of social systems as a defence against anxiety' from *Human Relations*, 1959, and Ian Suttie's *The origins of love and hate*, 1960, were also published about the same time. These studies of health professionals' denial of feelings, and their development of insensitivity to their own and others' distress, seemed to explain paediatric staff's resistance to the humane care for infants and children for which NAWCH was pressing (Chapter Four).

As well as reading psychoanalytic and psychological theories, NAWCH members drew on anthropology and on ethology, the study of animal behaviour. When members gave talks to parents' and community groups, they sometimes cited the plight of young monkeys separated from their mothers (Harlow and Harlow, 1961). These distressed monkeys were especially moving: it can be easier to understand messages that are not too close to home.

All these writers' emphasis on children's and other primate infants' constant need for their mother (or other stable mother-figure) and her role in protecting the child and mediating between it and the outside world, appealed to young mothers in the 1960s and 1970s. NAWCH's message was simple and direct. Many mothers responded to it, although they were probably unaware of NAWCH's theoretical underpinnings until they joined NAWCH. NAWCH's ideas resonated with their love for their children and their experiences of their own young children's behaviour. In addition, becoming a mother seemed to instil in some women a passionate wish to see all children protected from harm and injustice. Lay knowledge, lay ethical concerns, intense maternal feelings, the experiences of parents whose children had been in hospital and academic theory combined into powerful new knowledge. (Theories about babies' and young children's needs for their mothers are still contentious, and some people now regard psychoanalytic theories as socially coercive, convincing mothers to stay at home after the war because men needed jobs (Philips, 1988).) Although psychoanalytic theory is perhaps less fashionable today, it can be seen as a poetic metaphor for intense feelings that are difficult to name.

Nationally, NAWCH invited some paediatricians and paediatric nurses, whose practice in their wards NAWCH considered enlightened, to join the national NAWCH committee. NAWCH members' knowledge of parents' experiences in their local hospitals, together with this input from sympathetic or radical professionals, gave NAWCH a rich and wide body of knowledge, probably unique at the time (Elisabeth Hartley, member of NAWCH Executive Committee in the early 1970s, personal communication, 2008).

Locally, however, some NAWCH groups had great difficulty in persuading paediatric staff to accept unrestricted visiting. York NAWCH, for example, talked to the consultant paediatrician and the paediatric ward sisters (they listened); invited them to a showing of *A two-year-old goes to hospital* (they came); invited them to a day-long conference, with two distinguished pioneering (radical) paediatricians as speakers (they came). None of this had any effect. To show goodwill and serious intent, in 1969 NAWCH members, with Pre-school Playgroups Association members, raised money to build and equip a playroom in the grounds of the hospital and staffed it voluntarily themselves. An architect designed the playroom building and oversaw the building work, free; the Queen sent a donation; and the local Member of Parliament opened the playroom. Only after all that voluntary and community effort, did the consultant paediatrician agree to unrestricted visiting.

As a radical patient group, NAWCH was unusual in promoting a government policy. The Ministry of Health, as corporate rationalisers, here supported repressed interest holders, using NAWCH to oppose dominant interest holders more effectively than the Ministry could itself. (Corporate rationalisers were still weak in the 1960s, Chapter Two.) From NAWCH's earliest days, NAWCH's national committee members talked with civil servants in the Department of Health and helped draft official guidance (Belson, 2004). *Hospital facilities for children*, HM(71)72, which declared that visiting without restriction was essential, was so drafted (Belson, 2004). A year later, a NAWCH survey of all wards admitting children, found that 19% of children's wards had 24-hour access for parents; 32% had 10–15 hours; 33% had 7–9 hours; 14% had 4–6 hours; and 2% had 0–3 hours (Williamson, 1992). Between 1959 and 1991, the Department of Health issued five guidance circulars and NAWCH undertook five surveys. In the end, it took more than 30 years to secure unrestricted visiting in every paediatric ward in the UK (Williamson, 1992).

Looking back, it seems likely that the arguments from social sciences that NAWCH used had a greater effect in creating and sustaining members' commitment than in directly persuading local paediatricians and ward sisters to change their practice. Arguments from social sciences probably have less influence on health professionals than do those from

medical sciences. However, James Robertson, writing in 1988, believed
that campaigning by NAWCH, and the release to the public of his
films, created public sentiment as the main determinant of change
(Robertson, 1989). Journalists regularly used material offered to them
by patient groups, in radio, TV and newspapers (Council for Science
and Society, 1980). Isabel Menzies Lyth attributed changes in practice
to NAWCH, as well as to Bowlby and Robertson (Menzies Lyth,
1988b). Commitment from NAWCH members remained crucial for
many years, in the face of professionals' protracted resistance to having
parents present for particularly stressful times in their children's stays
in hospital (Chapter Six).

Today, this is ancient history. Parents, paediatricians, paediatric
nurses and managers take unrestricted visiting for granted. But
because NAWCH's story is over, it illustrates the enormous amount
of commitment, effort and time that is often necessary to change
dominant interest holders' practices and standards.

Knowledge from medical and scientific knowledge – RAGE – founded in 1991

RAGE, Radiotherapy Action Group Exposure, is a single-issue patient
group that draws on medical and physical science to argue for changes
to clinical standards and clinical research. It is like the AIDS activist
groups studied by Epstein, in that its members want to see effective
non-toxic treatments for their potentially fatal disease (Epstein, 1996).
But RAGE's membership has stayed in the high hundreds, that is, fairly
low compared with AIDS groups in the US; most of its members are
women; and its work, though judged by itself and by some oncologists
and radiologists to have successfully led to changed standards of
treatment, has been less well recognised (Hanley and Staley, 2006).

Some woman given radiotherapy for breast cancer in the late 1970s
and early 1980s, after the first warnings about radiotherapy fractionation
regimes and doses had been published in medical journals, began, after
a few years, to report to their doctors unexplained pain, loss of the use
of their arm, and other strange and alarming symptoms (Chapter Four).
When the women consulted their specialists, some of them denied that
the women's symptoms could be due to radiation damage, perhaps
because they did not know that. But other specialists knew, though to
their patients they denied it (Hanley and Staley, 2006).

◊◊ After surgery to remove a small breast lump in 1982, [this
patient] was given an appointment for radiotherapy. 'There was no

discussion on alternatives or possible risks ... about four months [after radiotherapy], I began to have very severe tingling all along my arm, followed by pain, then complete loss of feeling in the arm, even though the pain persisted.... I told the surgeon about this. He just barked, "You are absolutely A1" and rushed out of the room ... [though] he must have realised it was radiotherapy damage.' In 1986 she discovered, after a private appointment with a neurologist, that she had brachial plexus neuropathy. She also discovered that the hospital had acknowledged this to her GP. 'Nevertheless, the hospital kept denying to me that there was any problem at all. My request to see a radiologist was refused – "There was no point". The consultant almost reduced me to tears. I was "neurotic, arthritic" and it was "all in my mind". My husband was advised to "trade me in for one that doesn't moan"!!' (Hanley and Staley, 2006, pp 15, 16). ◊◊

Women gave RAGE many accounts like that one. In 1993 RAGE sent the Department of Health a list of 525 members who had developed injuries after treatment at the 53 radiotherapy centres in the UK (Hanley and Staley, 2006). Fifty-nine injuries had followed treatment at one centre; more than 20 at each of 5 centres; more than 10 at each of 12 centres; less than 10 at each of the rest (Hanley and Staley, 2006). These data showed that there were clusters of severe damage in some hospitals and in some years but not in others. This suggested that differences in total dose, or in fractionation regime or in technique, not in individual patients' different sensitivities to radiation damage, had been responsible (Sikora, 1994). RAGE approached the Department of Health, who (eventually) funded an audit of brachial plexus neuropathy by the Royal College of Radiologists, though RAGE had argued against the audit's being carried out by the College (Hanley and Staley, 2006).

Two radiologists from the College studied the medical records of 126 RAGE members and showed in 1995 that high doses of radiotherapy had increased the risk of damage (Bates and Evans, 1995). Margaret King, a member of RAGE and of the UK National Breast Cancer Coalition (Chapter Four), managed to obtain her radiotherapy records, studied them closely with the help of a radiographer friend, and read what she could find on radiotherapy (King, 1997). Dissatisfied with the College's report, she wrote a critique of it, published by the College in 1997, and sent by the College, like the first report, to all its members (RAGE, 1997). King criticised the report for errors in the data that Bates and Evans had abstracted from RAGE members' records; for failure to look at other studies; for obscurities in the text; for misleading presentations of some results; for expressing unsupported beliefs and assumptions; and for premature destruction of the data on which the analyses were based (RAGE, 1997). Unsupported assumptions included statements that brachial plexus neuropathy was rare; that it was possible to assume that because treatments were given accurately today, they had been in the past; and that patients would prefer the greater convenience of fewer, larger fractions to more, smaller fractions, in spite of the former's greater risk of damage (RAGE, 1997).

What effects RAGE's critique had on radiologists is hard to say. By the mid-1990s, radiologists had been alerted to the risks of radiotherapy to the breast and had changed their practice to reduce those risks (Hanley and Staley, 2006). Fractionation regimes and guidelines were progressively improved and doctors' understanding of the risks and benefits increased (Rodger, 1998). RAGE members felt that they had brought about this change; and some doctors agreed.

◊◊ 'Their achievements have been a massive improvement in British radiotherapy – people woke up in response to RAGE … There are no more cases of [brachial plexus neuropathy] due to radiotherapy, so they have achieved the long-term goal of changing practice. They may not see that they were responsible. That has been a major problem. The success of RAGE got no recognition from anyone – professional, political or legal,' said Dr Karol Sikora, oncologist (Hanley and Staley, 2006, p 93). ◊◊

◊◊ '… we did learn a lot from what happened to them, and because of that, patient care has changed for the better,' said Dr Michael Williams, radiologist (Whitcroft, 2007). ◊◊

Meanwhile, in response to concerns that RAGE had raised about wide variations in radiotherapy regimes, and its pressure to find the best fractionation regime through a clinical trial, the oncologist Dr John Yarnold set up a national clinical trial of different doses and fractionation regimes, to run from 1999 to 2008 ([The] START Trialists' Group, 2008). Its objective was to find out what standard practice should be. The draft protocol for the trial was immediately criticised by patient activists for using a total dose in one arm of the trial that was already known to be damaging; for lack of control over what parts of the chest were to be irradiated; and for letting the possible underfunding of radiology services influence the design (Rodger, 1998). That is, designing the trial partly to find the cheapest way of giving radiotherapy meant proposing doses thought by some radiologists and patient activists to be too high.

Margaret King criticised various points in the draft protocol of December 1995 (King, 1997). I list in italics some of her points, then suggest where the knowledge that she drew on to make them came from (see 'The sources of new knowledge', pp 74–80 above).

a. *The level of risk of severe complications deemed acceptable was too high*: experiential knowledge from her own damage and from other RAGE members' knowledge of the severe damage to other women; differences in opinion between lay people and doctors about what constitute acceptable levels of risk in relation to hoped-for benefits. (1 and 3)

b. *The information in the draft patient leaflet was 'inadequate, inaccurate, and misleading'*: her experience of not having been told enough before her treatment; her theoretical knowledge of what standards for patient information should be; her skill, as a solicitor, in checking the accuracy of the statements in the draft leaflet; lay ethical views about truthfulness. (1, 2 and 3)

c. *The lack of use of information from studies of different fractionation regimes already published*: informed lay knowledge about what is customary in research and her own reading of the research literature. (2 and 4)

d. *The optional use of an additional treatment field that would greatly increase the dose received by the brachial plexus, putting some women at an increased risk of damage*: scientific knowledge. (4)

e. *The idea that one fractionation regime could suit all patients, irrespective of the type of their tumour or its stage*: clinical knowledge. (4)

Breast UK (Chapter Four) also tried to emend the design of the trial, and asked Dr Yarnold to include one or two of its members in the trial's management group. That request was refused. Margaret King and Joyce Pritchard from RAGE, however, were accepted as independent observers, provided that they did not report back on confidential matters to any patient group. (Medical confidentiality allows doctors to consult their peers about research but does not allow lay people to consult theirs.) King and Pritchard secured some changes to the protocol, enough to enable Dr Yarnold to go ahead with the trial (Hanley and Staley, 2006). But RAGE and Breast UK continued to criticise the trial. Margaret King died of breast cancer in 2004.

◊◊ After the publication of the results of the trial in 2008, *The Lancet* published a letter from RAGE criticising the trialists' conclusion that larger, fewer fractions of radiotherapy (high dose) and smaller, more frequent fractions (low dose) gave the same results. The letter reminded readers that many women have disabilities after high-dose treatment in the 1980s that have only appeared many years later. Because radiotherapy injuries can be severely disabling 10, 20 or 30 years after treatment, the proposed 5-year follow-up was far too short. A companion study had not yet analysed patients' quality of life after radiotherapy; but the letter noted that the trialists reported that 'patients tend to score effects more severely' than physicians. (The letter refrained from commenting on that.) High-dose schedules might be cheaper; but many RAGE members would gladly have chosen daily low-dose treatment to avoid their present disabilities. The letter concluded that 'No final conclusions should yet be drawn about adopting high-dose schedules' (Carling et al, 2008). ◊◊

This example shows how difficult it is for patient activist groups to influence the design of clinical trials, though the AIDS groups Epstein studied seem to have been more successful (Epstein, 1996). But RAGE shows how radical patient groups can use new knowledge to judge whether clinical trials are scientifically and ethically acceptable. They can pick up weaknesses in the design and conduct of research. They can challenge and are ready to debate clinical and scientific assumptions and conclusions. They can compare researchers' data with those they get from their members. They can do 'quick and dirty' research that suggests lines of enquiry. They can oppose coalitions of dominant and corporate rationaliser interest holders, even if unsuccessfully, as in RAGE's objections to the Royal College of Radiologists carrying out an inquiry into its own members' work.

Apart from the clinical and scientific issues identified by RAGE, members' stories illustrated threats to patients' autonomy through concealing information and denying choice. They also showed the difficulties put in patients' way when iatrogenic harm is denied through ignorance or mendacity. Some RAGE women felt prolonged anxiety, constantly worried that their symptoms were caused by a recurrence of their cancer (Hanley and Staley, 2006).

Although radiotherapy techniques have been made safer since RAGE's early years, RAGE reported in 2007 that some patients were still being offered insufficient information about the possibility of severe, progressive and irreversible injuries, including death, from radiotherapy

(RAGE, 2007). The choice of whether to forego radiotherapy and have a different treatment or none was not always offered (RAGE, 2007). Patients were not always told that radiotherapy reduces local recurrence of breast cancer but seems to have no effect on survival (Goodare, 2007). Moreover, though fractionation regimes vary between centres, patients are not usually offered a choice of centres. Nor are they usually offered explanations of the rationales for the fractionation regimes and the techniques to which they give their consent, though those who know what to ask will be given an explanation (radiotherapy patient, personal communication, 2007).

Meanwhile, two other patient activists, former radiotherapy patients, have 'discovered', through using the 2000 Freedom of Information Act, that when 'untoward incidents' occur in radiotherapy, reports are not regularly sent to all other radiotherapy centres (Tylko and Blennerhassett, 2006). This was known to radiologists and to the Department of Health but no action had been taken on it (Tylko and Blennerhassett, 2006). To take no action on known risks to patients represses their interests (Chapter Seven, section on Safety). So there is a long way to go to improve radiotherapy services in the UK.

Conclusion

Radical patient activists' new knowledge, aligned with patients' interests and constructed from elements of knowledge from various disciplines set into a framework of experiential knowledge and ethical principle, is specialised knowledge. Medicine's knowledge changes as doctors begin to accept some parts of new knowledge, or at least begin to act in accordance with them. The radical criticism or idea becomes conservative (Chapter Three). But at first, new knowledge can seem either threatening or enlightening to dominant interest holders: probably radically inclined doctors see it as enlightening and conservative doctors as threatening (Chapter Nine). In creating new knowledge and using it to argue against dominant interest holders' coercive practices, with their avoidable harms to patients, radical activist patient groups contribute to lessening the repression of patients' interests for at least some aspects of healthcare. Similar processes, similar changes to society's knowledge, result from recognised emancipation movements. In creating and using new knowledge, radical patient activists are like other radical activists working to change things for the better by opposing oppression: they illustrate '... the expertise of activism, its courage, its persistence and its vision' (Fletcher, 2002, p 100).

SIX

Values, principles and standards

As one standard is achieved, it seems feasible and easier to set new ones.

(Christine Hogg, activist, and Jo Rodin, NAWCH member, 1989, p 16)

Introduction

This chapter looks at the principles that radical patient activists want to see guiding healthcare, principles expressed through standards of care. Patient autonomy is a fundamental value for activists and they identify new issues and press for higher standards in directions that support it. Activists work, that is, for standards that are emancipatory, progressively freeing patients from coercion and enlarging their opportunities for self-determination.

Standards

Healthcare is given through a multitude of ways of doing things, practices. Each practice can be given a prescriptive value, that is, made into a standard (Williamson, 1987). So standards are detailed rules about how to do things. Healthcare, consisting of complex series and networks of actions, can be thought of as guided or controlled by standards. Some are explicit, put into words either orally or in written or electronic documents. Some are implicit, guiding staff's actions, although not put into words. Some are latent, parts of complex actions, not yet singled out as separate actions and given values of their own. Practices or standards that do not exist in words can be as important as those that do: patients' interests can be repressed through lack of articulated standards (Chapter Two). Individual health professionals usually have a good deal of freedom to carry out their tasks as they wish (Strauss and Glaser, 1997). This enables them to do things that can benefit individual patients and their interests, like adapting what they say or do to each patient and to the situation that they are in. It also allows them to do things that can harm patients or their interests, either by commission or by omission, as the sociologists Anselm Strauss and Barney Glaser pointed out in 1970 (Strauss and Glaser, 1997).

The values attached to standards, explicitly or tacitly, can be taken from any field of knowledge or thought, from the highly technical to the everyday; from scientific research to feelings and intuitions; from academic arguments to beliefs based on personal experience (Williamson, 2000a). The values have usually been chosen by health professionals, sometimes by corporate rationalisers; that is both a mark of the choosers' dominance and a means of maintaining it (Chapters One and Three). What values they choose is partly a matter of practicality and feasibility, partly of power. The more powerful a profession, occupational or social group, the more freedom it has to choose values that suit its members' interests and that best sustain their ideological belief that they do good.

Ideas and insights

Radical patient activists work largely by trying to change certain standards or proposing new ones. But they do not do this at random. They act according to certain values and principles that we can call those of patient activism. *Values* are the worth of something, something worth having, in ethics, its intrinsic worth (Little et al, 1936; Brown, 1993). *Principles* are fundamental rules or guides to action (Little et al, 1936; Brown, 1993). Principles express truths, propositions or assumptions upon which other ideas and insights depend.

Patient activists have put their ideas, values and principles into words gradually. Their ideas did not arise fully articulated at the beginning of radical patient activism in the 1960s. This gradual creation and articulation of goals follows a common pattern for emancipation movements (Chapter One).

Ideas are born of putting together experiential and theoretical insights. The early patient activists picked up recurrent aspects of patients' experiences and feelings and joined them together or articulated them systematically in ways that fitted with the activists' insights and intuitions. These systematisations reflected and created sentiment, ways of thinking and feeling. Activists took some ideas and principles from other social movements and discarded others, further reflecting and creating sentiment that accorded with that they abstracted from experience. Intellectually, emotionally and politically, they began to build up new knowledge (Chapter Five). Blending their intuitively selected findings with eclectically chosen ideas that felt right, activists gradually came to think that certain principles regularly underlay the aspects of care they focused on and the positions they intuitively took on those issues. The principles they valued supported the ethical and political value, patient autonomy; but many activists did not make this connection at first. I follow this historic order in this chapter.

Principles

In the earliest years of patient groups, radical activists had three main sources to draw on for their work, for evidence and argument to support their intuitions and concerns.

1. Patients' recurrent reports of dissatisfactions and problems, including lamentations about inadequate information, restricted access when in hospital to their family and friends, biased hearings of their complaints, lack of respect from staff.

2. Early activists' own intuitive choices of what to look for on visits to hospitals and how to judge what they looked at.

    ◊◊ Activists challenged restricting visiting times for child patients in hospital; restricted visiting for elderly patients in hospital; excluding the baby's father from its birth; preventing children from visiting their parents or grandparents in hospital. ◊◊

3. Sets of standards published by national professional bodies or by the Department of Health, like *Improving geriatric care in hospital*, published in 1975, and *The organisation of the in-patient's day*, 1976 (British Geriatric Society and Royal College of Nursing, 1975; DHSS and Welsh Office, 1976). Activists and health professionals have long taken ideas for standards from each other, especially when both draw on wider social values. Activists find it useful, in any case, to cite official and professionals standards, since doing so gives greater authority to what they say.

Gradually, activists came to see that specific principles seemed to determine what practices, standards and issues they saw as significant and worked to change. (In the examples in 2, the principle was support.) So the principles themselves, as they became identified, could be used as part of the argument put forward. That was a major advance. It gave coherence and direction to activists' work. Since the principles reflected the values held by the wider society of which the health service is part, it also gave activists' work legitimacy.

The principles that radical activists drew out of their experiences, discussions and reading over the first 20 or so years of the patient movement, from the early 1960s to the late 1980s, were: choice, information, access, respect, equity, shared decision making, safety, support, representation and redress (Williamson, 1992; 2003).

Choice, information and support were probably the first principles to emerge in the early radical patient groups like AIMS and NAWCH (Chapter Four). Social movements appropriate some ideas and principles from other social movements (Phil Brown et al, 2004). Other movements' ideas can reinforce a group's own ideas or put into words their half-articulated thoughts. Information, respect and greater control over medical decisions were principles of the early women's movement in the US (Zimmerman and Hill, 2000). Information, respect and shared decision making were principles of the civil rights and patients' rights movements in the US (Annas, 1998). Access, information, choice, safety, representation and redress were principles of commercial consumerism (Potter, 1988). Equity was foreshadowed by Alford with his term 'equal healthcare advocates' (now patient representatives, advocates or activists) for those who sought high-quality healthcare for everyone (Alford, 1975).

Social movements in the US were especially good sources of principles. The women's health movement in the US in the late 1960s was the first movement to challenge modern medicine, predating the patients' and the disability rights movements (Zimmerman and Hill, 2000). Quality of care was its main goal (Zimmerman and Hill, 2000). Similarly, higher standards of care were the goals of early radical patient groups in the UK. The American Civil Liberties Union published *The rights of hospital patients* by the lawyer George J. Annas in paperback in 1975 (Annas, 1975). Some of those rights were aspirational standards, not legally enforceable. Again, the emphasis was on standards of care. Moreover, at the time, American medical ethics was about 10 years ahead of British medical ethics (Dr Arthur Dawson, Canadian cardiologist, personal communication, 1996). This was significant because medical ethics and radical patient activism have some values and principles in common.

Radical activists give their own meanings to some of the principles they appropriate. Attributing new or special meanings to words is part of the creation of new knowledge (Williamson, 2008a). The next chapter gives radical activists' definitions of words like equity and safety. Radical activists' appropriation of some ideas does not mean that they accept all the tenets of the donor group or social movement (Chapter Five). Thus, some activists in the 1980s and 1990s accepted the term 'consumer' although they did not accept the commercial aspects and implications of commercial consumerism. Consumerism's market origins and market ideology seemed irrelevant, as the NHS was free at the point of delivery. To activists (and I was one) 'consumer' simply seemed a useful term for patients and those who aligned themselves with patients, a category for whom there is still no accepted term (Williamson, 1992). But it was easy for governments, professionals and managers to confuse commercial consumerism with patient activism. (Indeed, the term patient activism was seldom used then.) Some professionals tend to see consumerism in healthcare as selfish, unethical and even anti-social. So this confusion was, and remains, unfortunate.

Thinking about their principles gave activists the inductive insight that those principles supported a fundamental value, patients' autonomy. In the examples under 2, where the principle was support, the radical challenge was to professionals' coercive control over patients and relatives, and the value, still latent in the 1960s and 1970s, was autonomy for patients and for those who normally support them, their parents, partners, relatives and friends.

Patient autonomy

Personal autonomy is a basic value in western societies (Jensen and Mooney, 1990). Autonomy can be defined in various ways. But individuals' freedom to act, within the law, without coercion by other people, must be expressed or implied in the definition (Jensen and Mooney, 1990). Beyond that definition, people disagree over whether individuals can sometimes act independently of other people or whether individuals are always interdependent with other people, known and unknown, and cannot act truly alone. Women's 'caring connection with others', attributed to them as part of their moral life, seems to contrast with the individualistic and separate sense of moral identity attributed to men (Gilligan, 1982; Chanter, 2006, p 75). But this distinction between men and women may be too sharp (Chanter, 2006). In any case, in some sense, we are both alone and in communities with others all our lives. So an expanded definition of patient autonomy should allow for feelings of interdependency, of responsibility and of altruism, as well as of independence and of self-concern. The following definition, a composite of three sources, does:

> *Respect for patient autonomy means upholding patients'*
> *opportunities and abilities to control as far as possible the impact of*
> *illness or disability on their lives in ways that accord with their own*
> *moral and cultural values, their responsibilities to themselves, their*

> *families and their communities, and their interests as they define them.*
> (Olszewski and Jones, 1998; Williamson, 2003; Edwards,
> 2003)

This definition covers patient autonomy for preventive medicine, immunisation, screening and palliative care, as well as for diagnosis and treatment. It covers patients with acute illnesses and people with long-term medical conditions who want to get on with their lives as best they can (Levenson and Joule, 1999). It covers patients with limited or variable capacity to act autonomously on their own, like young children or people with severe learning disabilities. Even when patients' autonomy of action is constrained or reduced by illness or frailty, their autonomy of thought and will should be respected (Weale, 1988).

In everyday patient care, patients can make autonomous choices of dependency. "You choose, doctor", or "do what you think best", can constitute autonomous choices, based on private analysis of the situation (how experienced is this clinician? what is his reputation?), not on feelings of dependency. Or patients may choose to rely on relationships of trust and engagement with the professionals caring for them, rather than to make independent choices (Edwards, 2005). The essence here is freedom from coercion.

Autonomous choices of dependency, however, can raise difficult issues. One is the power of dominant interest holders to set discourses and agendas in such a way that repressed interest holders are unaware that their interests, as they would define them, are threatened (Lukes, 2005; Chapter Two). Then patients may be trusting their clinicians' advice blindly, from covert coercion.

Another problem is that some people have an internal locus of control and believe that their decisions and actions determine the state of their health; other people have an external locus of control and believe that the state of their health is determined either by powerful other people, like health professionals, family and friends or by chance, luck or fate (Wallston and Wallston, 1982). Patients with internal loci of control can recall information about their illness and its treatment better than those with external loci of control (Lavelle-Jones et al, 1993). Better-informed patients seem to make a better recovery from surgery than patients who are less well-informed or less interested in the details of their surgery (Lavelle-Jones et al, 1993). If patients with internal loci of control generally have better outcomes than those with external loci of control, all patients should probably be encouraged to contribute to clinical decision making, even if they feel reluctant (Michael Wang, professor of clinical psychology, personal communication, 2008).

Some hospitals and some professionals, in fostering dependency and in taking control over patients' actions, are probably better suited to patients with external loci of control than to patients with internal loci of control. This has ethical and therapeutic implications. It also has political implications, for patients with strong internal loci of control are more likely to be radicalised, if professionals are overbearing, than patients with external loci of control.

The relations between freely chosen dependency by patients with strong internal loci of control, dependency due to patients with external loci of control and dependency due to covert coercion need study. All three are probably among the complex factors that allow patients as a social group to be dominated by other interest holders (Chapter Two).

Autonomy and the core principles

Exactly when the connection between patient autonomy and the core principles emerged explicitly from activists' unspoken consciousness is uncertain and probably varied, perhaps widely. It became clear to me by the late 1980s (Williamson, 1992). In the early days, patient autonomy was probably little recognised as the key value for radical patient activism for at least three reasons, already touched on.

1. Patient activists' responses to what they saw as low standards of care were at first intuitive. Intuition is an immediate apprehension of something without the intervention of a process of reasoning (Brown, 1993). It is based on experience, feeling and knowledge. It is not irrational. But the reasons for the judgements it prompts are not always easy to put into words. Intuition is like poetry, where meaning can go beyond words.

2. Radical patient groups were young. They had to observe different patterns and standards of care, listen to what patients said, hear different reactions from health service staff and managers to suggestions, criticisms and requests, exchange views with colleagues, read books and papers, before their theoretical insights could emerge.

3. Some of the concepts patient activists needed to interpret their experience and give shape to their thoughts were not yet in common discourse (Chapter Five). Members of social movements can seldom invent every concept they need. As well as appropriating concepts from other social movements and academic sources, they can take them from the very social groups whose assumptions

and actions they challenge. Patient autonomy began to be written about by medical ethicists and so became salient for doctors in the 1970s in the US, in the 1980s in the UK (Annas, 1998; Furness, 2003). Only then did the concept become easy for patient activists to come across.

Patient autonomy and medical ethics

The concept of patient autonomy links radical patient activism and medicine. The exact meanings each attributes to it are likely to be different. But there is a common core of meaning that makes it possible for patient activists to appeal to doctors to act in accordance with their own professed values and to accept practices and standards that support rather than undermine patient autonomy (Chapter Nine). The principles, too, are supported by many doctors (Smith, 2003). Where doctors are likely to differ from radical activists, and indeed from each other, is in the degree to which they accept the expression of the principles through specific standards, that is, exactly where they draw the boundary between what is acceptable to them and what is not (Smith, 2003). Radical activists will want policies and standards to give the strongest possible expression of the principles: full information, not selected bits of information; access to up-to-date treatment for all patients, not just for some; as many choices as possible, and so on. Doctors will think that certain limitations are necessary or desirable, though different doctors will want different limitations. Many conflicts over specific issues, whether to include or omit something in patient information leaflets, for example, turn on questions of degree. There is seldom open disagreement over the principles themselves. But doctors and patient activists will want to see standards for information, access, redress, etc. on their terms, not on the others'. So conflict is almost inevitable.

Table 6.1 is a list that the anaesthetist Dr Andrew Smith drew up of 16 practices for which anaesthetists could offer choice to patients. He ranked them in order of their contentiousness to his consultant anaesthetist colleagues, that is, in order of their probable reluctance to offer them to their patients. Radical patient activists would welcome them all.

Table 6.1: Practices ranked in order of contentiousness to anaesthetists

Things which probably don't matter to anaesthetists either way
- Which arm or hand to have the IV (intravenous) cannula inserted into (a cannula is a device that lets fluids to be given directly into a vein)
- Whether or not to have a sedative pre-medication
- How to travel to theatre (walk, wheelchair, trolley)
- Whether or not to watch the operation

More contentious
- Whether to use a local anaesthetic cream to reduce the pain of cannulation (having the cannula inserted)
- Whether to have injection or mask (for gas) for the induction of general anaesthesia (all other things being equal)
- Role in choosing the type of pain relief post-operatively
- Leaving jewellery (especially a wedding ring) on

More contentious again
- Encouraging patients to enquire about the status and experience of the anaesthetist
- Allowing adult patients to have a friend or relation accompany them into the anaesthetic room
- Allowing the patient to choose whether to have local or regional or general anaesthesia (unless one or other is clinically necessary)
- Offering the PILs for the drugs to be given (PILs are the manufacturers' patient information leaflets which must be included in every packet of drugs)
- Trusting patients to stick to the fasting time for clear fluids

And further again ...
- Offering patients a copy of their anaesthetic record
- Offering patients copies of the relevant protocols for the procedures to be used
- Encouraging patients to ask if a particular form of care is available in a particular hospital (eg a high-dependency unit for post-operative care)

Source: Andrew F. Smith, personal communication; Smith, 2003

Dr Smith's heading for non-contentious practices, 'Things which probably don't matter to anaesthetists either way', indicates the emotional investment that doctors have in the standards they prefer to work to. Even the choices for the first three practices are not always offered. (The fourth is likely to be opposed by some surgeons.) Anaesthetists may find treating all patients in the same way more convenient than offering choices; or oppose choices because they shift some power to patients (Smith, 2003).

Similar lists could be drawn up for principles, practices and standards in every specialty. The lists would change over time, some high standards for choice, information, support and so on dropping off the lists as they became incorporated into routine practice and were no longer issues. New issues would join the lists as practices and standards previously taken for granted came to be questioned, and so became contentious.

Identifying new issues

Smith's table suggests how practices and standards become issues, become contentious: just putting them into words can draw attention to their potential for conflict. Someone questions a hitherto routine part of practice, a taken-for-granted standard. That someone may be a patient, a health professional or a patient activist. An issue is defined as a point in question, a matter of contention, a point that is ripe for decision (Little et al, 1936; Brown, 1993). This definition is legal in origin, but it suggests that issues are always potentially controversial.

The number of actions that are taken every day in healthcare is very large and each one has, or could have, a value attached to it, a standard. When a practice or standard becomes an issue for activists, they may seek to replace the standard's current value by another one. Or they may seek to abolish a practice altogether. Or they may seek to break down a practice into component practices and give each one a value, that is, set a standard for it. Or they may seek to articulate a new standard for a new practice, particularly when professional practice changes or new technologies bring new ways of doing things. Identifying issues in practices and standards that are taken for granted by professionals, patients and patient activists is akin to consciousness raising in recognised emancipation movements. Radical patient activists and radical professionals are more likely to identify new issues than are conservative ones, who mostly accept the status quo (Chapters Three, Eight and Nine).

◊◊ AIMS and the National Childbirth Trust (NCT) published a charter, a set of desired standards, for ethical research in maternity care, in 1997 (AIMS and NCT, 1997). They drew attention to women's vulnerability and powerlessness when in hospital and to their responsibility for their babies as well as for themselves. One of the charter's standards was that the practice of asking for women's consent for research when they were actually in labour should stop. Proposals for research should be discussed with pregnant women well before childbirth (AIMS and NCT, 1997). ◊◊

Here the standard 'seek women's consent to research' was broken down into temporal components. Telling women about research and seeking consent at one particular time should be abolished and replaced by another time.

As this example suggests, patient activists sometimes want to guide, even control, clinicians' behaviour just as much as corporate rationalisers do. They are not in as powerful a position to do so (Chapters Two and Ten). But they are not always without influence of their own. Or they can join forces with corporate rationalisers over some issues, just as they can join forces with clinicians over others. The tripartite play of interests and alliances among interest holders is a complicated, never-ending dance in which the dancers change partners at irregular intervals, as well as dancing some steps solo, 'in an elaborately choreographed ballet – with the dancers constantly changing partners and adopting new formations as the setting of the drama changes' (Klein and Lewis, 1976, p 132). (This metaphor matches Alford's depiction of three sets of interests and interest holders, published a year earlier, Chapter Two.)

Activists' sense of direction and sequences of standards

Activists' sense of direction, by which they judge some standards as 'low' and others as 'higher' or 'high', developed early in radical patient groups. Standards that prescribed more information, a more thorough investigation of complaints, greater support and so on were deemed higher by activists than those that prescribed less, other things being equal. The higher the standard, the greater its direct or indirect support for patient autonomy, the more liberating from others' coercive control. This sense of direction, combined with new knowledge, determines what issues activists identify and try to resolve through changes to practice and through standards that they define as higher.

Activists' sense of direction also helps them to predict what further changes to standards they and patients will want to see. The changes to standards and patterns of care that activists work for can be thought of as a sequence of steps towards an ultimate goal, greater respect and support for patient autonomy, as well as better treatment and care in general. Once a new standard is accepted and begins to be implemented, the next step towards the goal often becomes possible. Like activists in recognised emancipation movements, radical patient activists are seldom satisfied.

Sequences may be vertical, a series of ever-higher values for the same practice, like the steps of a staircase. Or sequences may be lateral, with higher standards spreading sideways, like interconnecting rooms on the same floor of a house. The highest value for a standard may be visible from the first, from the bottom of the staircase or from the first room. Or it may be so distant as to be unimaginable at first.

◊◊ *1. A vertical sequence, the highest standard visible from the first.*

The highest standard for parents' access to their children in hospital, free access for 24 hours a day, was enunciated by the Department of Health and Social Security in 1966, in HM(66)18. It was reinforced in 1971 in HM(71)22, which said that visiting without restriction was essential. It was reinforced again in 1976 and 1991 (Williamson, 1992). NAWCH surveys showed that in 1951, 23% of children's wards allowed no parental visiting; by 1962, most wards allowed between half an hour and five hours. By 1969, there was unrestricted visiting in the daytime, 5%; no visiting in the mornings, 25%; other hours, 30%. By 1973, 24 hours, 19%; 10–15 hours, 32%; 7–9 hours, 33%; 4–6 hours, 14%; 0–3 hours, 2%. By 1983, 24 hours, 49%; other, 51%. In 1986 NAWCH resurveyed the wards that were worst in 1983 and found 24 hours in 85%, other hours in 11%, and restrictions on the day of surgery in 4% (Williamson, 1992). By the end of the 1990s, all children's wards had unrestricted parental visiting, though some adult wards that admitted children and some neonatal units did not (Peg Belson, personal communication, 2008). ◊◊

It took parents' requests and complaints, and repeated requests and arguments by local NAWCH groups and by some community health councils (Chapters Five and Eight) to bring about fully unrestricted visiting throughout the UK.

◊◊ *2. A lateral sequence, the highest value visible from the first.*

Once unrestricted parental visiting was beginning to be accepted and introduced into paediatric wards, parents told NAWCH that they were being prevented from remaining with their child for some procedures and routines. NAWCH then took up further issues relating to the principle of support: whether parents could stay with their child during ward rounds, during diagnostic procedures and in treatment rooms, for the induction of anaesthesia and recovery from it. Each move to allow parents to remain with their child was resisted by health professionals, sometimes for years. Most are now accepted (NAWCH, 1990). The Royal College of Anaesthetists has not adopted parents' presence for the induction of and recovery from anaesthesia as a national standard. But the Association of Paediatric Anaesthetists accepts it as good practice (Crean et al, 2003). ◊◊

◊◊ *3. A vertical sequence, the highest value, the one at the end of the sequence, the top of the staircase, too distant to be visible at the beginning.*

In maternity units in the 1950s, husbands were allowed to be with their wives for the first stage of labour only, and then sometimes only during visiting hours. AIMS and other maternity care patient groups set about trying to change that. By the 1960s, husbands or partners were (sometimes) allowed to be present for spontaneous deliveries; by the 1980s for instrumental deliveries; by the 1990s, for caesarean sections under regional anaesthesia (Williamson, 1987; Royal College of Obstetricians and Gynaecologists, 2001). By the 2000s, the issue had become whether partners could be present for elective caesarean sections under general anaesthesia (Seymour, 2004). (It is not in question for emergency caesarean sections, where every minute may matter to the outcome.) Here the argument turns not on support for the unconscious woman, but on the father being able to witness the baby's birth and to welcome him or her into the world. The idea arouses strongly antagonistic feelings in some obstetric anaesthetists. Others allow it (Andrea, 2001). ◊◊

Each of these steps over the last 50 years was attained through individual women's requests and complaints and through action by maternity care patient groups. Each successive step was fraught with anguish and anger. Each successive step required repeated arguments and appeals to professional bodies, to the Department of Health, to sympathetic midwives, obstetricians and managers. Probably the early AIMS activists who pressed for the first step did not envisage the partner's presence for caesarean sections. It would have been almost inconceivable, 'too glaring a prospect' (Chapter One).

Sequences like these provide evidence that radical patient activism takes emancipatory actions, incrementally opposing the status quo. Similar sequences exist for information, for shared decision making and so on; but sequences for support are easier to trace because visiting times and rules are explicitly stated in hospital leaflets.

Professional and institutional resistances to new ways of doing things are fairly well understood (Sisk, 1993; Wootton, 2006). Where a change would result in some loss of power to professionals, resistance can be strong and protracted (Wagner, 1994). Then the cost of that resistance in upset and misery can be high, for professionals as well as for patients and patient activists. Recognised emancipation movements evoke resistance and anger, too; and painful, though often erratic, sequences of social change are probably typical of the process of emancipation. Restricted parental visiting for child patients in hospital may now seem as remote as this sequence:

◊◊ No education for most girls; universal primary and secondary education for girls but no university education for women; university education for women but not to study medicine; women allowed to study medicine. ◊◊

Defining exactly where a sequence starts and ends can be difficult. But activists are sustained by their sense of dynamic progression towards new vistas for healthcare.

Principles together support autonomy

So far, I have looked at each principle on its own. But principles interact in the sense that a standard for a single practice can affect how far other principles can be met. If patients are not informed that other treatments for their condition exist, they cannot choose between them or protect their safety by avoiding risks they would rather not take. That is obvious; but the ramifications can be extensive. The next example illustrates this. I started from the principle of information; but I could have put the other principles (in italics) first.

◊◊ Autologous blood transfusion is the transfusion of the patient's own blood, collected some days before elective (planned, not emergency) surgery and used, if needed, instead of donor blood. In the late 1990s and early 2000s some hospitals provided the service to clinically suitable patients, others did not (Howard et al, 1992). Some of the latter hospitals did not give patients the National Blood Service's leaflet, current in 2002, about blood transfusion because it mentioned autologous transfusion as well as explaining about transfusion in general (National Blood Service, 2002; consultant haematologist, personal communication, 2002). Withholding this national leaflet undermined other principles, not just *information* (Williamson, 2005). *Safety* was threatened because autologous transfusion is safer than allogenic (donor) transfusion: autologous transfusion cannot introduce viruses like HIV, or prions like new variant CJD, into an uninfected patient, nor cause immunological reactions (Holland, 1999). Most haematologists would prefer it for themselves (Chapman, 1999). *Shared decision making* was vitiated because it depends on doctor and patient sharing all relevant information. Here the doctor knew something relevant, the local clinical policy, and the patient did not. Similarly, *respect* for patients was lacking, because what was known to doctors and managers was deliberately kept from patients. *Choice* was denied, because patients could have chosen to forego elective surgery or to seek it at another hospital or to ask about other methods of conserving their own blood (also mentioned in the leaflet). *Equity* was undermined because disadvantaged patients were less likely to know about autologous transfusion independently of the hospital than well-informed patients. To be in a position to ask questions and make requests, disadvantaged patients needed the leaflet more than advantaged ones did. *Access* for patients to autologous transfusion was prevented because some hospitals that did not routinely offer autologous transfusion did provide it on request. (Or, if patients had known, they could have chosen to seek treatment at another hospital.) Asking for something is one of the few ways in which individual patients can take some responsibility for the quality of care of their local services. Even one request, if granted, can set a precedent that removes the restriction for other patients. It is a pleasanter way of bringing about change through *redress* than by making a complaint. *Representation*, too, was hindered, for unless patients were aware of the deficiency in provision, they could not take political action to highlight it on behalf of other patients (Williamson, 2005). ◊◊

◊◊ When this patient told the others in her hospital ward that she had had an autologous transfusion, they wished that they had had one with their own blood instead of with donor-blood (Stubbs, 2001). ◊◊

Principles reviewed in the next chapter

In the next chapter, the ten core principles that patient activists believe should guide healthcare are discussed. Examples are taken from current or recent issues over which patient activists and many doctors or corporate rationalisers hold or have held conflicting views. Standards of care rouse strong feelings in professionals and in patient activists. Seeing conflicts over standards in terms of principles makes such conflicts seem less like a multitude of erratic and hostile challenges to professionals and institutions and more like steps on the way to progressively helping professionals and corporate rationalisers make healthcare more congruent with social values and patients' interests.

Patients vary in how much information, shared decision making, support and so on they want, either absolutely or at different stages of their episode of patienthood (Chapter Seven). Patients' right to decline the partial or the full expression of a principle is taken for granted in the next chapter. Ideally, each patient and clinician should arrive at a shared understanding of what the patient wants, as the episode progresses. But mismatches between patients' and clinicians' understanding of what, for example, shared decision making means, and cross-purposes in their interactions with each other, are probably common (Edwards and Elwyn, 2006; Entwistle, 2006).

Other principles

Other principles could be added to the ten core principles in this and the next chapter. They could be entirely new ones. Or, more likely, they could be new principles to give separate emphasis to ideas subsumed under the existing principles.

◊◊ *Continuity of personal care* for the patient from the same clinicians is becoming more important as corporate rationalism splits the care of patients between various health workers. Continuity of personal care can be subsumed under *safety* or under *respect*; but it may need to be emphasised by making it into a principle in its own right. ◊◊

Who judges how important particular principles are, who identifies new principles, and when, depends on many social factors. As the patient movement matures, we can expect to see two fundamental principles of recognised emancipation movements, justice and equality, made explicit. These two principles are discussed in Chapter Eleven.

Coda

Powerless individuals want autonomy, and radical patient activists want it for patients (Chapter Two). The first group to advocate personal autonomy in patients' decisions about healthcare was the women's health movement in the US (Zimmerman and Hill, 2000). Now some patient groups, patients and doctors subscribe to the idea of patient autonomy (Chapter Ten). But it has seldom been a published primary goal of radical patient groups. That may be because they take it for granted or because the groups' strengths and effectiveness lie primarily in the detailed evidence and argument they can give about the harms and goods they identify, not in their abstract aspirations. But there comes a time for declaring that patient autonomy is a primary goal of radical patient activism, using an expanded definition, like the one in this chapter, that includes patients' concerns and responsibilities for other people as well as for themselves.

SEVEN

The ten principles

Introduction

This chapter discusses the ten principles named in the last chapter: respect, equity, access, information, safety, choice, shared decision making, support, representation and redress.

Respect

> *What upsets me most is when the public are saying "what we need is respect and dignity". If we are not doing that, what the hell are we doing?*
> (Lord Darzi, surgeon, 2008, in Whitworth, 2008, p 5)

Respect comes from the root to look back at, to regard, and means to esteem or honour (Brown, 1993). In healthcare, *respect means seeing patients as morally equal to oneself as well as treating them with courtesy and consideration* (Fried, 1974). The lawyer Charles Fried said that, ideally, each patient and each healthcare professional should see himself or herself as an autonomous person, bound to others, known and unknown, in a network that is expressed through moral equality, autonomy and mutual respect (Fried, 1974). This ideal can be captured through the idea that patients are people whose capabilities and responsibilities should be respected and supported, not inhibited or undermined (Chapter One).

> ◊◊ 'I do not want to enter the surgery and leave my personhood and capacities outside the door. How can I then use my resources to aid my recovery?' said a cancer patient in 1988 (Jolley, 1988). ◊◊

Patients' laments that professionals fail to respect them 'as a person', or to see them 'as "real" people', are as plangent today as ever (Chapter One; Bates, 2001; Help the Aged, 2008). Lack of respect for patients seems endemic in the health service, especially in NHS hospitals. Here are a few of the many points that patient activists, patient groups and Community Health Councils (Chapter Eight) have taken up in writing or discussion with the Department of Health or with trusts. Most are long-standing or recurrent.

Environment

Privacy: from being overheard when talking with staff or visitors.
Comfort: wards and waiting areas with windows and views; comfortable furniture.
Protection: from unnecessary exposure to distressing sights or to staff's frivolous or heartless talk; from negative or threatening notices; from unnecessarily harsh lighting.
Information: easy access to library or electronic information.

The institutionalised way things are done

Security: control over who can enter a ward or department and when; clear name badges for staff; explanations of nursing and multidisciplinary teams' memberships.
Privacy: knocking on doors before entering.
Safety: minimal pre-operative fasting times.
Dignity: out-patient waiting areas not like cattle markets; patients summoned by name, not by numbered tickets; decorous clothes for staff; patients only addressed by their first names with their permission.

Personal behaviour

Responsiveness: listening and responding to what patients say; offering explanations of what will happen; avoiding baby talk; agreeing to patients' wishes whenever possible.
Self-control: not talking to each other when making the patient's bed; not avoiding relatives who wish to see a senior doctor or nurse.
Ethical conduct: not summoning students to look at unusual 'cases' without that patient's consent; not 'consenting' patients instead of seeking their consent or refusal.

Some changes to physical facilities are hard to bring about quickly. Harsh design in the first place, and the persistence of apparently easily changed practices and habits, seem to reflect deeply negative views of patients. It looks as if, at some level of dominant interest holders' consciousness, perhaps an unconscious level, patients are felt to be inferior beings, not worthwhile people (Chapter One).

Equity

> *... the aim of a life can only be to increase the sum of freedom and responsibility to be found in every [person] and the world. It cannot, under any circumstances, be to reduce or suppress that freedom, even temporarily.*

(Albert Camus, philosopher, 1961, p 240)

Equity means treating people with fairness and justice (Brown, 1993). *In healthcare, it means treating patients with the same needs equally in respect of those needs.* Healthcare professionals and patient activists agree so far. After that, their interpretations of equity are apt to diverge. Health professionals tend to level down. They tend to want to deprive all patients of opportunities that for some reason cannot be offered to or taken up by every patient who might benefit from them. Activists want to level up (Williamson, 2003).

◊◊ In the 1940s, nurses justified preventing parents from visiting their children in hospital daily on the grounds that some parents were too poor to travel every day (Vaizey, 1959). Twenty years later, NAWCH dealt with this problem by working to secure funds or help with transport for parents who needed them (Belson, 1981). ◊◊

◊◊ In the 2000s, an eminent pathologist wrote in an article about the introduction of new laboratory tests, 'It is surely not acceptable for patients in one part of the UK to benefit from a new test which is denied to a patient in another' (Furness, 2007). A patient activist response was to put this the other way round, 'It is surely not acceptable for patients in one part of the UK to be denied a new test which benefits patients in another part of the UK' (Williamson, 2007b). ◊◊

◊◊ In the 2000s, innovative birthing centres and services like one-to-one midwife care were ended in some parts of the UK because there were not enough midwives to offer them to every pregnant woman (Nadine Edwards, personal communication, 2008). ◊◊

Levelling up offers at least some patients something that might benefit them, rather offering all patients nothing. As well as increasing some patients' opportunities and freedoms, it has pragmatic advantages.

Patients collectively would benefit, if unequal treatment were used as a 'real life' experiment in which the experiences of both groups were, with their consent, kept under close review, so that the advantages of the treatment, if demonstrated, could be extended to all patients.

The issue of equity is made more difficult because professionals sometimes have punitive attitudes towards patients who try to secure good care. 'Informed' or 'active' patients are often seen as selfish, middle-class, *Guardian* readers, happy to seize priority over other, more deserving, patients. Professionals can write about them bitterly or resentfully (Greenhalgh and Wessely, 2004). That 'selfish' patients seek for themselves no more than they would wish for all other patients, and that their requests can have a social and political value, leading to improvements in provision or in standards of care, presumably does not occur to them.

Levelling down undermines justice for patients as a social group because it represses the interests of patients collectively; inhibits new developments and extensions of good practice; and permits erratic and sometimes covert rationing. In that, it is coercive. The levelling-up approach works in the opposite direction. Limited resources for healthcare in rich countries result from governments' choices (Delamonthe, 2008). That, with many doctors' acceptance of those consequences and their toleration of deficient systems for the organisation and management of resources, is a mark of the overall repression of patients' interests.

Access

Access means a way or means of approach (Brown, 1993). *In healthcare, it means putting opportunities for reaching some desired aspect of healthcare within reach of any patient who might need it.*

Access is closely related to equity, the equitable access to some healthcare good. Some aspects of access, like long waiting times for out-patient appointments, are artefacts of a specific healthcare system's arrangements. The same is true of equity. The conditions for access and equity can be adjusted according to policy and to resources, though structural or political aspects may make this hard.

Access is also like equity in that socially, educationally, physically or mentally disadvantaged patients may need more help in reaching and using what might benefit them than advantaged patients do. That is taken for granted when hospitals and GPs' surgeries provide ramps and handrails. But it extends to things like offering access to further information and help in interpreting it or help in asking for and interpreting test results and medical and nursing notes.

Access and equity should prevent discrimination against categories of patients. Women are sometimes offered less treatment than men (Chapter Three). Older patients may justifiably fear that their age alone, rather than their overall health, will preclude them from being offered effective treatment (Wilkie, 2003). Positive discrimination on clinical grounds can be right. But access should otherwise be equitable.

> ◊◊ At an 8am out-patient anticoagulant clinic for taking blood to monitor the effects of warfarin regimes, patients on their way to work were seen first, even when they arrived after those not in paid employment. A patient's protest to the trust's director of the service resulted in no change (patient, retired GP, personal communication, 2008). ◊◊

Patients may willingly give priority to other patients, just as people do for each other in ordinary social life. But patients' altruism, not staff's dictates, should decide.

Information

> *Lucidity. The patient has a right to know all the relevant details about the situation he finds himself in ... Denial of lucidity is a sufficient condition for a relation of dominance, and that in itself is a violation of right.*
> (Charles Fried, 1974, lawyer and medical ethicist, p 101)

> *Secrecy is part of the fabric of medicine ...*
> (Charles Medawar and Anita Hardon, social activists, 2004, p 71)

Information is knowledge or instruction that can be communicated (Brown, 1993). Patient activists' position on information is simple: patients should have easy access to full information about the situations in which they find themselves. This will usually include access to the information that the professionals caring for them have, because patients consider that professionals are their most important sources of information (National Health and Medical Research Council, 2000). But some patients also need and want independent sources of information and opinion (Coulter et al, 1999).

Information has potential goods for patients, including:

- **Therapeutic.** The therapeutic benefits of information are hard to identify precisely. But accurate information and compassionate explanation can help patients to understand their predicament; remove groundless fears; help them to cope with anxiety; help sustain their confidence in their ability to manage their relationships with other people, including the professionals looking after them; and, for those with internal loci of control, help them to feel in some control of their treatment and care and its outcomes.

- **Ethical.** 'Full' information is information that avoids the least suggestion of deceit or any coercive withholding of what the patient might want to know (Chapter Two).

  ◊◊ A pathologist at the Royal College of Pathologists asked a radical patient activist how much he should tell parents about post-mortems. She replied "everything". He unfolded successive levels of detail: she reiterated "everything" to each (personal observation, 1997). ◊◊

- **Political.** Patients need information in order to consider how their interests might be supported or threatened by the treatment and care that will be provided, or not provided, for them. Then they can take individual or social action that may benefit themselves and other patients (Chapter Six).

These goods of information are clouded by complex problems and conflicts of interests.

1. Questions about what the patient wants to know or not to know at any stage of an encounter with healthcare and questions about how the patient can decide what he or she wants to know, without knowing what that might be, complicate discussions about patients' 'information needs'. Patients' psychological strategies for coping with anxiety can either limit or increase their wish for information (Leydon et al, 2000). Information can in theory be made accessible in hierarchies or layers, each hidden from the patient until he or she chooses to access it (National Health and Medical Research Council, 2000). But practical ways of doing this are neither common nor satisfactory.

2. Patient activists want patients to be offered more information than 'ordinary' patients usually think that other patients will want.

◊◊ Some 'ordinary' patient members of a working group composed of patients, patient activists and anaesthetists, writing patient information leaflets together, wanted risks played down, with no details in the texts (Rollin, 2003). The patient activists wanted all known risks included, while the anaesthetists' views were in between (Rollin, 2003). ◊◊

Individual patients usually have to rely on their personal views to judge what other patients want. Patient activists draw on wider knowledge. They know that a harm that may be unimportant to some patients can be devastating to others. "If only they had told me beforehand" is a familiar lament after a harm has occurred (Chapter Four). Activists know that many patients who say beforehand that they do not want to hear about risks change their minds if they are told about them: the possible harms are usually less terrifying or less common than they had feared (Parroy et al, 2003).

◊◊ Even after things had gone well and no harms had occurred, most patients in one study who had wanted not to hear about the risks of possible harms said afterwards that they would have liked to have discussed them more fully when making the decision to have the treatment or procedure (Moore et al, 2002). ◊◊

So patient activists' views can conflict with those of 'ordinary' (non-activist) patients. This can be hard for professionals and managers to understand and can make it difficult for them to decide which view, if either, to accept.

3. Some clinicians tend towards offering little information. Doctors have inherited a medical culture in which beneficence, the wish to do patients no harm, can lead them to conceal upsetting information from patients (McCullough, 1988). Beneficence as an ethical value was salient long before patient autonomy became ethically important, and 20 years ago some doctors used it to override patient autonomy (McCullough, 1988). Remnants of this sort of beneficence, and of its brother, paternalism, remain. But withholding information without the patient's expressed wish to hear no more is potentially coercive (Chapter Two).

4. Clinicians, like everyone else, usually act from several motives, not just one.

◊ ◊ The radical activist Madeleine Wang argued the case for offering patients information about all the known risks of anaesthesia, taking inadvertent peri-operative hypothermia (pathological coldness during or after an operation) as an example (Wang, 2007, p 2233). She had 'had a scrap' with a surgeon, whose arguments against telling hinged on 'pandering to the needs and wants of the white middle class, [the use of] resources, trees and rainforests, causing undue worry to patients about matters of which they have little control or choice' (Wang, 2007). Wang's arguments hinged on patient autonomy. 'Healthcare has progressed from a place where information was a mere conduit to patient compliance to one of assisting concordance and beyond, where patients will in some circumstances choose to forgo anaesthesia and surgery because the risks for them are too great a burden to bear' (Wang, 2007, p 2234). ◊ ◊

Anaesthetists' letters in the *Bulletin of the Royal College of Anaesthetists* in response included 'I do not know of anyone who actually does inform the patient of this risk'; 'I ask [patients] if they want to know about other complications' and '[n]o one in 20 years has ever taken me up on this'; patients can look things up on the internet; and offering full information would be impractical and too time-consuming (Kestin, 2007, p 2368). Also, anaesthetic patients are not fully autonomous because they are too anxious and fearful to be rational and an approach should balance autonomy with paternalism (Stimpson, 2007).

Arguments based on clinicians' personal experience, like those based on patients' personal experience, must be respected; but they must be put into wider contexts. Clinicians' arguments can seem as unconvincing to patient activists as activists' arguments can seem unrealistic to clinicians.

5. Some issues are more problematic to clinicians than to activists. Should patients be told about accidents that happened to them but of which they were unaware and that probably will not harm them? Activists base their 'yes' on research and on their view of the basis of trust between patient and clinician.

◊ ◊ In a questionnaire study, 92% of 246 patients but only 60% of 48 ophthalmologists thought that the patient should always be told if an unintended injury, which had a 10% chance of impairing vision in that eye, occurred during cataract surgery (Hingorani et al, 1999). ◊◊

Some clinicians base their 'no' on the impracticalities of telling patients; difficulties of knowing what counts as too trivial to matter; and possible harm to the doctor–patient relationship (Heneghan, 1999). Patient activists ask what the patient would feel if he or she were not told, but found out (Williamson, 1999b).

6. Another controversial issue is whether patients should be told about treatments that might benefit them but that are not provided by the NHS locally. Patient activists think they should. Corporate rationalisers and some clinicians tend to think they should not (Milne et al, 2000). Silence supports covert rationing and conceals the limitations of the health service (Marcus, 2007). Some clinicians stay silent from beneficence (Firth, 2007). Others think that if the treatment of one group of patients is to be compromised for the benefit of another group, that must be made clear to those patients; doctors' duty of veracity requires that (Spry et al, 1993).

Controlling what and how much information patients had access to was the main way in which doctors preserved professional dominance in the past (Stimson and Webb, 1975). Today the internet has weakened that control (Vaitheeswaran, 2009). Questions about how far patients can find reliable information on the internet; whether they should be expected to search for it, and how they can be helped to, if they need help; and what is the legal and ethical minimum information that patients must be offered in person by their doctors before they treat them, that is, for informed consent, arise (Skene and Smallwood, 2002). But the internet can provide a rich source of knowledge and of the benefits of that knowledge (Shaw, 2009).

Information begins to lift repression from repressed interest holders by enabling them to consider their interests and voice their views. Conflicts between patient activists and clinicians (and corporate rationalisers) over information are likely to persist, though some of the issues will probably change.

Safety

> *For decades, the medical profession itself has documented high levels of error, far higher than other industries tolerate.*

(Lawrence L. Weed, physician and specialist in medical informatics, 1997, p 231)

Safety means protection from hurt or injury, freedom from danger (Brown, 1993). But much healthcare involves exposing patients to the risk of the occurrence of harm in return for hoped-for benefits. Only the patient can decide what risks he or she is willing to accept in relation to the hoped-for benefit; acceptability is a personal matter (Herxheimer, 2005). So safety in healthcare needs careful definition.

Safety in healthcare means avoiding avoidable risks and discussing with the patient unavoidable risks (Williamson, 2003). Clinicians are free to undertake high-risk procedures, provided that the patient understands the risks and gives consent, or, if the patient is not in a position to do so, the procedure is judged in his or her interests, as in General Medical Council guidance for all patients (General Medical Council, 1998; Williamson, 2003). There must be no bias in giving patients information about risks and benefits.

◊◊ Women who ask for a home birth are usually given a list of the risks of harms to which they expose themselves and their babies (Anon, 2007/8). Women who choose to have a hospital birth are not given a list of the risks of harms they run in hospital, though for healthy women at low risk of complications in childbirth, the risks are greater there (Anon, 2007/8). ◊◊

Avoidable risks of harm

The distinguished medical expert in the quality of healthcare Dr Donald Berwick said that avoidance of risks is not always intelligent or conscientious (Berwick, 2003). The will, the ideas or the implementation may be lacking (Berwick, 2003). Clinicians tend to be blind to their own unsafe practices, though when they are patients or relatives, they notice those of other clinicians (Berwick, 2003). Medical culture and hospital systems can mean that the same dangerous practices and common mistakes are made over and over again (Flynn, 2006; Uddin, 2006).

◊◊ The Healthcare Commission found that 40% of trusts in England had not complied fully with basic standards of safety in 2007 (Coombes, 2008). About 10% of patients admitted to hospital in the UK are inadvertently harmed by the care they receive (Department of Health, 2001). ◊◊

Reviews, bewailings and resolutions to do better abound. Whatever the causes, whatever the relative contributions of systems' failures and of individuals' failures, the perpetuation of avoidable risks dramatically reflects the repression of patients' interests.

Unavoidable risks of harm

Here conflicts of view circle round the issue of how much to tell patients in advance about the risks of harms from any procedure, including diagnostic procedures and treatments. General Medical Council guidance says that 'any serious or frequently occurring risks' should be explained (General Medical Council, 1998, p 4). 'Serious' and 'frequently occurring' can mean different things to different people. But even without that problem, patient activists and doctors seldom agree on whether all known risks should be mentioned (see the section on Information). Patient information leaflets (PILs) state the known risks of medicines, though the relevant PILs are not always offered to patients, either in hospital or before they take up their GP's prescription. Information about the risks of non-operative procedures, like intubation, is not always easily available.

Patients' own safety

How far patients should engage in helping to secure their own safety is also controversial. Offering patients the referral guidelines for diseases they fear they might have could reduce the possibility of their GP missing a sign or symptom that turns out to have been significant.

> ◊◊ A proposal from the Patient Liaison Group of the Royal College of General Practitioners that the college should encourage GPs to show patients who were worried about the possibility of breast cancer the national referral guidelines, *Guidelines for referral of patients with breast problems* (Austoker et al, 1995), was rejected (personal observation, 1997). ◊◊

Offering patients the management protocols for their chronic diseases and the treatment protocols for their acute diseases could let them check that the steps were carried out (Williamson, 1995). As guidelines apply to populations of patients and may be unsafe for some individual patients, it is especially important that patients discuss them with their doctor (Woolf et al, 1999). It would also meet the wishes of some patients.

◊◊ Elaine McColl, 'an informed consumer and an advocate of evidence based medicine', wanted to see the guidelines or protocols for the management of her glaucoma (McColl, 2005, p 155). She found a comprehensive guideline, with almost 600 references. But she did not know whether her ophthalmologists had consulted it. There was no lay summary of it, nor reference to patients' concerns (McColl, 2005). ◊◊

These ideas are far from new, but they are not yet generally accepted.

Other patients' safety

Patient groups and individual activists think that patients can sometimes contribute to safety for other patients. Professionals and corporate rationalisers tend to resist each specific proposal, at least at first.

When a scheme for providing doctors with Yellow Cards to mail to the regulatory agency (now the Medicines and Healthcare products Regulatory Agency, MHRA) to notify it about possible adverse reactions to drugs was introduced in 1964, patients were deliberately excluded from taking part directly (Inman, 1999). 'It is unlikely that patients would be able to judge what events were drug reactions ... not helpful for them to report directly to the Committee in lay terms what their doctor should be doing as part of his professional responsibility' (Inman, 1999, p 101). The letters of public-spirited patients who wrote nonetheless to the agency about possible adverse reactions (side effects) were simply put to one side (member of MHRA staff, personal communication, 2004).

It soon became apparent that doctors habitually under-reported the adverse reactions caused by the drugs they had prescribed (Blenkinsopp et al, 2006). By the mid-1990s, MIND (a mental health patient organisation), social reformers and patient activists were calling for patients to report their suspicions direct to the regulatory authority (Blenkinsopp et al, 2006). In 2004, the government, following a recommendation from an official report on the Yellow Card Scheme, decided to introduce reporting by patients, 'patient reporting' (Steering Committee for the Review of Access to Yellow Card Data, 2004).

◊ ◊ A working party of patient activists, doctors, pharmacologists and MHRA staff, chaired by the radical patient activist Patricia Wilkie met monthly from November 2004 to October 2005 to design the contents and format of a yellow card for patients to send direct to the MHRA. After protracted discussions, the MHRA staff and the activists reached agreement on many points. But the MHRA refused to flag up black triangle drugs (drugs that require special vigilance once launched on the market) or off-label drugs (drugs prescribed for a condition or age group for which the drug has not been licensed by the MHRA). The patient activists thought that patients needed to be alerted to these drugs, both for their own safety and because their reports on suspected adverse reactions to such drugs could be especially valuable. ◊ ◊

Analysis of published research from countries where patient reporting had been established showed that the quality of patients' reports was similar to that of doctors and other health professionals (Blenkinsopp et al, 2006). In addition, patients reported some new possible adverse effects that healthcare professionals had not reported, or patients reported them more quickly (Blenkinsopp et al, 2006).

Published discussions of the proposed scheme disclosed disturbing assumptions:

1. The professionals and civil servants who opposed patient reporting thought that it could divert attention from 'the more important … reports from health professionals' and might be used by patient campaigning groups 'to create a signal', that is produce biased evidence against specific drugs or reflect consumers' 'preconceived notions of the bad effects of medicines' (Steering Committee for the Review of Access to Yellow Card Data, 2004, pp 71, 72). So they assumed that patients' reports would always be less valid than professionals' and that patient groups might behave dishonestly.

2. A pilot scheme asked patients to report via nurses on a telephone helpline, rather than directly to the MHRA. But nurses weeded out (that is, suppressed) some of the reports (Steering Committee for the Review of Access to Yellow Card Data, 2004). The idea that nurses or other health professionals can act as proxies for patients is common, in spite of its implausibility.

3. Some civil servants talked of giving patients the 'right to report' direct to the MHRA (Choonara, 2004). The idea of a 'right' is curious

since, in most other situations, it would be a person's duty to report an adverse occurrence, a traffic accident, say.

These points suggest how little patients' observations, capabilities and motives were respected. Thinking ill of other social groups helps dominant interest holders to repress their interests and restrict their actions (Chapter One). Then those repressed interest holders cannot easily show dominant interest holders that they are wrong. Corporate rationalisers and health professionals seem willing to tolerate patients contributing to safety only as a last resort.

◊◊ Doctors are poor at complying with standards on hand washing or on using alcoholic gel rubs, though these precautions prevent the spread of most infections (Gawande, 2004). So some hospitals now tell patients 'do not hesitate to remind doctors, nurses ... to clean/wash their hands before attending to you' (York Hospitals NHS Trust Infection Control Team, 2004). ◊◊

Falling back on patients for some important task is like falling back on women to replace men in factories during the Second World War. Such moves can be liberating. But they are a mark of how far freedom to contribute responsibly to society has been denied.

Choice

The ideal of a human life to which the physician ministers is an ideal of a life fully, lucidly lived, a life whose major events and constraints are accepted and internalised into the structure that a free and thinking man creates of that life.

(Charles Fried, lawyer and medical ethicist, 1974, p 99)

To make a choice, or to choose something, is to take it by preference to all other things that are available and that could have been preferred (Brown, 1993). Most people continually make choices about trivial and important things. The German 19th-century philosopher Nietzsche thought that a worthwhile life is something we must each create for ourselves, as an artist creates a work of art (Nehamas, 1957). We create our lives through our choices, even when we are constrained by social structures. The necessities forced upon us by chance or through other people's actions give us new opportunities for choices as well as new constraints upon our choices. The more serious and intractable the situation we find ourselves in, with a life-threatening illness or as an inmate in a harsh or confusing setting, the more important choices become. They retain for us symbolically, and to some extent in reality, some control over life as well as still expressing and creating the self (Spriggs, 1998). Even premature babies can indicate their preferences (Alderson et al, 2005).

Choice refers to the choices patients make on their own or with the advice of their relatives and friends. People can make some choices outside the medical model and medical control. Childbirth, the menopause and dying can be treated as natural, biological events or phases in life, socially influenced, but not needing medical surveillance or treatment (Conrad, 2000). Some complementary medicine treatments are also non-medical. (But if they fail to work, the medical model can be tried.) Conversely, people whose problems fall outside the medical model and have not been defined as illnesses may want to have them so defined and treated (Zavestoski et al, 2004).

Choice can be separated conceptually from shared decision making with a clinician, but they can overlap in practice when the patient makes a choice from knowledge or beliefs or intuition and the clinician agrees to it.

Different treatments for the same disease or condition can be based on different scientific premises, be experienced differently and carry different risks and benefits, short-term and long-term consequences. Choices that could be offered are many. Most have a history of conflict and some are still not offered routinely. They include:

- *Choice of treatment setting*: of home or hospital for childbirth; home, hospice or hospital for dying; GP surgery or hospital out-patient department for diagnosis and minor treatment; a specific hospital for a specific diagnostic procedure or treatment.

- *Choice of practitioner*: of GP; of hospital specialist; of anaesthetist as well as of surgeon; of midwife; of care manager; physiotherapist, and so on.

- *Choice of diagnostic procedure*: of antenatal scan or no scan; of electronic continuous foetal monitoring by a machine or of intermittent monitoring by a midwife.

- *Choice of mode and scope of treatment*: surgery, radiotherapy, chemotherapy for cancer; no treatment but careful surveillance (some cancers, high cholesterol levels); extent of surgery – mastectomy or lumpectomy for breast cancer; radical or non-radical surgery for colon cancer; mode of delivery of treatment, for example, of fractionation regime in radiotherapy; drugs given orally or intravenously; intention of treatment, for example, curative or palliative; natural childbirth or interventional childbirth.

- *Choice of non-clinical aspects of care*: whether an adult patient can have a relative or friend with him or her while waiting for the induction of anaesthesia; whether the patient should be present at a clinical team meeting when his or her case is discussed; whether the clinician or the pathologist should tell the relative about the post-mortem findings.

- *Choice of whether to enter a clinical trial*: whether local or further afield, if the patient meets the requirements of the trial's design.

Some choices have to be asked for by patients who happen to know about them.

◊◊ A scientist made a graph of his exponentially rising PSA levels (prostate specific antigen in the blood, a marker of possible prostate cancer) but biopsies found no malignancy. Another scientist suggested that he ask his consultant to refer him to a unit where a new form of diagnostic radiology was being developed. That showed a small cancer, found on a new biopsy to be just on the verge of becoming dangerous (Gleason stage 7) (patient, personal communication, 2006). ◊◊

◊◊ A patient with breast cancer asked her consultant to arrange for the oestrogen receptors in her excised breast tissue to be tested, a test then becoming standard good practice but not yet offered in that hospital. The test predicts whether women will benefit from treatment with anti-oestrogens like tamoxifen (Elledge and Osborne, 1997). He refused (patient, personal communication, 1996). ◊◊

Choice expresses a patient's authentic preference only when the patient has access to all the relevant information about all the courses of action that could be taken in respect of the situation the patient is in. This requirement brings us back to issues of information and equity.

Although patients are offered more choices now than in the past, there have been backslidings. Some primary care trusts have rescinded patients' customary 'right' to be referred to a consultant of their and their GP's choice (dismayed patients, personal communications, 2009).

Some professionals see choice for patients as trivial. Or they see the government's efforts (admittedly ambiguous and contradictory) to increase patients' choices as ploys to destabilise the NHS; or to control doctors through patients; or as party political points (Radcliffe, 2004). Though these points about official policies are probably partly true, the value of choice as a principle is unaffected.

Shared decision making

Power is the ability to take one's place in whatever discourse is essential to action and the right to have one's part matter.

(Carolyn Heilbrun, feminist and literary scholar, 1989, p 18)

Some decisions, like whether to visit the GP or what steps to take in an emergency with an unconscious patient, can be taken only by the patient or only by the doctor. But many decisions can be taken by patient and doctor (or other autonomous healthcare professional) together, sharing information and ideas with each other and arriving at a plan of action that both can accept (Tuckett et al, 1985). Shared decision making is often envisaged as a process in which patients contribute knowledge of their own bodies and their hopes, values, feelings and ideas, and doctors contribute evidence from research and their clinical knowledge, experience and judgement (Stewart et al, 2003; Coulter et al, 2008). But this division between patient and clinician is too sharp. The patient may have acquired relevant clinical knowledge from various sources.

◊◊ Patients with chronic diseases sometimes know more about them than most professionals (Levenson and Joule, 1999). Their knowledge is different from doctors' knowledge and, in their view, can be superior to it (Macintyre and Oldham, 1977). ◊◊

◊◊ Some guidelines advise patients to remind their doctor to follow the guidelines, 'your doctor may have forgotten about [them]' (PACE Angina Project, nd, p 4). ◊◊

The doctor, too, will have feelings, preferences and interests, for no clinical decision can be separated entirely from its personal and sociopolitical environments. Rationing and doctors' double role as agents of the state and of the patient are ethically problematic (Klein, 1993). So are financial incentives to doctors to take some courses of action rather than others (Chapter Two). Lack of candour about the situation that doctors find themselves in can justifiably erode patients' trust in them.

◊◊ An unmarried woman in her sixties, sexually inactive, received three peremptory letters summoning her to attend her GP's surgery for a cervical smear: 'an appointment has been made for you ...'. Had the summons been framed as a population measure, she might have consented. Presented as a benefit to her, she presumed it was motivated only by her GP's desire for financial reward, and felt insulted (patient, personal communication, 2002). ◊◊

So *shared decision making can be defined as a process in which doctor and patient bring all their relevant knowledge and other resources to the problem for which the patient seeks the doctor's help.*

Shared decision making entails an exchange of information, values, reservations and experience between doctor and patient, including the doctor's recommendation about the course of action he or she thinks best, if the patient invites that (Quill and Brody, 1996).

◊◊ A pioneering study in the US, in which approximately equal numbers of patients with chronic conditions and doctors worked together to identify attitudes and behaviours that facilitated shared decision making, emphasised the need for patient and doctor to develop a relationship of mutual respect, trust and empathy (Lown et al, 2009). Both patient and doctor explore the patient's feelings and preferences. Both contribute information and seek information and advice from sources outside their relationship (friends, clinical colleagues, the internet). Both share power and control, each sometimes deferring to the other. Mutual influence can help patient and doctor arrive at a course of action that neither might have thought of on their own. In the end, the preferences of each are integrated into a decision that both agree with; or they agree to disagree and the doctor honours the patient's decision. The doctor acts as the patient's advocate in helping him or her to circumvent institutional constraints, if necessary, while the patient takes responsibility for acting on the plans they have agreed (Lown et al, 2009). ◊◊

In the UK, a more negative approach seems to prevail. Much has been written about some patients' and some doctors' disinclination to engage in shared decision making (Sinclair, 2008). Also discussed have been:

doctors' wish to retain the power of controlling the patient in the consultation through setting the agenda and through deciding what course of action should be taken (Elwyn et al, 2000); the skills both doctors and patients will need to negotiate courses of action (Elwyn, 2006); practical difficulties, like lack of time (Kravitz and Melnikow, 2001); whether respect for patient autonomy can leave the patient with too little guidance from the doctor (Sokol, 2007); and the whole idea as an 'idealistic construction' of academics (Elwyn, 2006).

Meanwhile, as these debates go on, surveys show that many patients say that they were not as much involved in making decisions about their care as they wanted to be: 32% in primary care, 48% in hospital care, in a national survey in England in 2006 (Richards and Coulter, 2007).

◊◊ Research showed that staff in neonatal intensive care units seldom discussed proposed courses of action with parents, even about matters well within parents' competence to help decide, like when they could take their baby home (Alderson et al, 2006). ◊◊

In addition, patients continue to tell patient groups about decisions made without discussion with them, sometimes against their expressed wishes (Ryder, 2007/8). So theories and hopes about shared decision making, however it is defined, are well ahead of its practice.

From patient activists' perspective, one of the important aspects of shared decision making is its potential for reducing coercion in healthcare. The bias in the next example would be incompatible with shared decision making.

◊◊ General practitioners admit that they sometimes bias the information they offer patients, in order to gain their consent to one course of action rather than another (Rees Jones et al, 2004). ◊◊

Coercion is expressed through policies undisclosed, referral and treatment guidelines not shown to patients; patients deemed ineligible for treatment without truthful explanation; beneficial treatments not mentioned (Chapter Two; Williamson, 2005).

Confusion about what shared decision making means and vicissitudes in putting it into practice repress patients' interests and expose them to experiences that they may judge oppressive.

Support

> *... needless to say the visit of your spouse plus or minus other sundry relations and friends is often the highlight of the day.*
>
> (B.T. Marsh, doctor who had been a patient, 1987, p 909)

> *... attachments provide security ...*
>
> (Joan Woodward, 2008, psychotherapist, p 152)

Supporting people means preventing them giving way, holding them up, bearing weight for them, maintaining their value (Brown, 1993).

Being with someone to whom one is emotionally attached is the most direct and probably the most effective way of being supported at times of anxiety and stress, provided that the person wants that support. Separating patients from relatives and close friends removes that prop, just when patients may need it most. In addition, it can increase professional and institutional control over patients in various ways, including by potentially undermining their sense of their own value and significance to other people (Williamson, 1992). It also prevents relatives from witnessing or intervening in poor care. The early campaigners in radical patient groups seeking to secure support for child patients and for women in labour knew that (Williamson, 1992).

These early campaigns started the long and unfinished haul to secure unrestricted or open visiting for all patients in hospital. Although now most hospitals have visiting patterns that enable patients to receive some support from relatives and friends, each successive gain has a history of intense and often protracted conflict (Chapter Six). Flexible visiting, visiting by people of the patient's choice at times that suit patient and visitor, was officially recommended in 1976 (DHSS and Welsh Office, 1976). It is not yet widely implemented in the UK. The highest possible standard is to permit visiting by relatives and close friends at all times. This has been introduced in a few hospitals in the US; visitors (and staff) are asked to keep noise low between 7pm and 7am (Frampton et al, 2008). But pockets of serious resistance remain.

◊ ◊ Some neonatal intensive care units limit parents' access to their babies, even though babies tend to have better sleeping and breathing patterns when their parents touch them (Alderson et al, 2005). ◊ ◊

Backslidings also occur.

◊◊ York Hospitals Trust, having introduced visiting times of 2–8pm in 1985 for adult acute wards, reverted in 2007 to two periods, 3–4.30pm and 6.30–8pm. The reasons given were infection rates and the bad behaviour of visitors and of a few patients (Patient Advice and Liaison Services staff, personal communication, 2008). These reasons are the same as they were 40 years ago. ◊◊

Professionals' and corporate rationalisers' power to limit the support that patients are able to receive from people closely connected to them is a sad reminder that patients are an oppressed social group.

Representation

> *[Patient representatives] may be the only members of a [professional–patient working] group that are able to stand up effectively to the views of professionals that might otherwise prevail.*
>
> (Margaret Martin, independent healthcare consultant, and Lucy White, anaesthetist, 2003, p 147)

Representation is the action of presenting a statement about something that is intended to convey a particular view and influence other people's opinions or actions (Brown, 1993).

One might expect the representation of repressed interest holders' views or interests to dominant interest holders to be fraught with difficulties and resistances. It is. Professionals and corporate rationalisers tend to misunderstand what representation is, sometimes confusing it with representativeness or statistical typicality. (Although patients' 'representativeness' bothers them, they seldom question their own 'representativeness'; this is a double standard, Chapter Nine). They may fail to distinguish between patients and the public or between views and interests. They may find it difficult to accept that patients and patient activists have different kinds and levels of knowledge from which to make statements. They may make no distinction between, or confuse, radical and non-radical positions or be unsure how to judge the validity of what patient activists say. They are sometimes reluctant to explore how much patients can contribute to topics other than direct patient care. Misunderstanding and confusion indicate underlying conflicts of objectives (Alford, 1975). But the patient movement has not always clarified these matters, either.

Who can speak for patients' interests is affected by three sets of factors.

1. Healthcare political alignment: radical or conservative

This was discussed in Chapter Three. What patients or patient activists representing the interests of other patients say has to be judged by the evidence and arguments they use, just as it has for people representing other interests (Williamson, 1998). A quick way to judge whether a stated position is radical or conservative is this: radical views are more likely than conservative views to work in the direction of increasing patients' opportunities to act autonomously. This applies also to radical and conservative clinicians (Chapter Nine).

2. Activists and non-activists

Activists are patients who are trying to change some aspect of healthcare and so are politically engaged with other social groups in healthcare. They may be patients acting on their own, or active members of patient groups, or patient representatives or advocates. Non-activist patients are 'ordinary' or 'real' patients not trying to improve healthcare. (As this book is mostly about radical activism, I usually use 'activist' as shorthand for 'radical activist', except when I add the word 'conservative' to activist.)

Radical activists in social movements create and lead 'oppositional consciousness' as they synthesise ideas from various sources, draw attention to injustices and mobilise support (Mansbridge, 2001a). Non-activists select and use some of the ideas that activists articulate (Mansbridge, 2001a; Chapter Ten). This is how radical ideas spread (Chapter Eleven). Non-activists are always more abundant than activists, so their spreading of the ideas they select is crucial to any emancipation movement. But there is a time lag during which many non-activists and conservative activists continue to support dominant interest holders' interests and views on specific issues, long after radical activists have opposed them.

3. Kinds and levels of knowledge and experience

Individual patients can speak from their own experience. They can watch what goes on, and notice what does not go on; identify new problems in hitherto accepted practices and standards; and make requests, suggestions or complaints. That can influence patterns or standards of healthcare, either directly through professionals or indirectly through the patient movement.

◊◊ A 10-year-old boy asked to see his colon, excised because of ulcerative colitis. The pathologist who showed it to him and his parents decided thereafter to invite all children who had had surgery for bowel disease to see their excised colons (Domizio, 2008). ◊◊

This boy, in making his request, potentially increased the opportunities and freedoms of other patients to make choices and to understand their own clinical situation more fully. But patients can speak only from their own experience. They cannot speak for other patients' interests.

◊◊ A group of young people were asked what information about anaesthesia should be offered to patients of their age due to undergo surgery. They wanted the information to be brief (Madeleine Wang, personal communication, 2008). By wanting to limit the information offered, the young people acted against other young patients' opportunities and freedom to understand choices, patterns of care and risks in anaesthesia. ◊◊

This example shows why patient activists are wary of professionals' and corporate rationalisers' propensity to rely on the views of small numbers of non-activist patients. In general, both conservative and radical patient activists think that only findings from valid samples of populations of patients, or from patients meeting together in focus or other purposeful groups to discuss issues and standards of care, can be taken as valid recitals of patients' views. Findings can indicate both majority views and important minority ones. Majority views that would increase patients' freedom please radical activists. But they are not disheartened by those that do not; they know that the spread of radical ideas takes time.

Patient groups can represent the interests of other patients like themselves. Activist members of patient groups know what those patients' experiences and judgements are; what standards of care in the specialty should be; what policies and practices are controversial; what new treatments or procedures are in the offing; what kinds of treatment and care patients say they would like. Their specialised knowledge is their strength (Chapter Five). Their weakness is, as with all specialists, a tendency to idiosyncratic views (Williamson, 1998; 2007c).

All relevant patient groups should take part in any consultation that seeks to give voice to patients (Williamson, 1998; 2007c). Some categories of patients are not covered by any patient group, and then research into their experiences and views may have to be commissioned.

Patient representatives or *advocates* have often gained experience in several patient groups. They have a general and abstract knowledge of the interests all patients have in common (Williamson, 1998; 2007c). They can explain the 'patient perspective' on issues like confidentiality, consent, information and trust, where professional definitions and views tend to differ from those of patients. They, and activist patient group members, are likely to discern any hidden threats to patients' interests in healthcare professionals' and corporate rationalisers' policies. They are often used to working with healthcare professionals, especially doctors and midwives. Patient advocates' weaknesses are that they may lack both patients' recent, first-hand experience and patient group members' familiarity with the specialty and with controversial issues in it.

One or two patient advocates should take part in any consultation. Professionals or corporate rationalisers making appointments to working, liaison, advisory or steering groups should be aware of the radical–conservative dimension in patient advocates, as well as in themselves and their colleagues (Chapters Eight and Nine).

These three categories of patient overlap. For most consultations, several patients, a member of all relevant patient groups and one or two patient advocates should take part. Only that way can the weakness of each kind of patient be overcome. The exact composition of a group intended to speak for patients' interests should depend on the nature and level of the consultation (Williamson, 1998; 2007c). Again, commissioning research into the experiences and views of samples of specific sorts of patient may be necessary.

Confusion about representation and lack of knowledge about how to seek the views and understand the interests of patients as a social group gives dominant interest holders reasons for disregarding their views. Giving full, or sometimes any, expression to the principle, representation, is distant.

Redress

Redress gives protection against the powerful.
(BBC Radio 4, 10 April 2008)

Redress is reparation or compensation for a wrong or for a loss resulting from that wrong (Brown, 1993).

Devising complaints procedures for healthcare that patients and professionals both think fair is extremely difficult. The differences in power between them and the assumptions that historically underpin systems for redress make it so. Patients or relatives can readily believe that the system is biased against them. They can feel at the mercy of doctors. Reciprocally, doctors' awareness of the ever-present possibility of being complained against can make them feel that they are less powerful than patients (pathologist, personal communication, 2004). Both complainants and those complained against have high stakes in the procedure and in its outcome.

Over the years, patient-aligned bodies, including the Association of Community Health Councils in England and Wales (ACHCEW), the National Consumer Council and the Patients Association, have tried to get complaints procedures reformed (Gilbert, 1995; National Consumer Council, 1996; Robinson, 1999). Over the years, the Department of Health has introduced successive reforms to the system. Each has failed to satisfy all parties. 'The current system seems to serve nobody's interests,' wrote Hilary Gilbert in 1995 (Gilbert, 1995, p 36). That remains true. In 2001, the Department admitted that it had not succeeded (Department of Health, 2001). It knows that complainants feel that current procedures are 'still not responsive, accessible or independent enough' (Department of Health, 2001, p 27). It has promised to reform the system again (Rose, 2008).

Reformers believe that certain principles should underlie all complaints systems. These should be: natural justice, fairness, thoroughness, access, simplicity, speediness, effectiveness, responsiveness and user friendliness (Birkinshaw, 1994; Nicol, 1999). Thoroughness is important in all hearings of complaints or appeals (Williamson, 1985). It can uncover aspects of a case that were hidden under the surface. Biases can lurk in procedures, as well as in how they are carried out. Biases are sometimes not even hidden.

◊◊ On a General Medical Council panel hearing a complaint against a doctor, a lay member was told to take "a lay perspective" not "a patients' interests perspective". The medical members were not instructed to take "a non-doctors' interests perspective" (lay member, personal communication, 2006). ◊◊

When a complaint is upheld, redress in money is not offered. For that, complainants must go to law. But complainants often want not money but an apology and a commitment from the individual or institution to prevent the same thing happening to other patients (Robinson, 1999). Although doctors are disinclined to believe in patients' altruism, *the reformation or correction of something wrong* is a secondary meaning of redress (Brown, 1993).

Redress is a fallback for patient autonomy, for the self-as-moral-agent. It can assure patients and relatives that, however terrible the events that prompted them to complain, they are not powerless to try to change things for the better.

EIGHT

Conflict and schism

... from the beginning, [the second wave of the women's movement] was not unified: the agenda was various, the disagreements multiple, the discourse diverse – there was no golden age of harmony and purpose. The radical edge was like a magnet, both drawing and repelling the moderate middle, fuelling the energy for change.

(Susan Krebs, feminist writer, 1997, p 87)

Introduction

The patient movement is fragmented and split, and so politically weak (Chapter Three). Conflicts among patient groups and between individual activists make it difficult for groups to work together as a unified movement. This chapter suggests that the radical–conservative dimension, the differences between radical and conservative convictions, lies behind some of these conflicts. Some conflicts seem so recurrent and so intractable as to suggest schism in the patient movement.

Convictions and schisms

The lack of an ideology in the patient movement means that patient activists working to improve patient care or called on to speak for patients' interests in advisory or policy-making official bodies have to rely chiefly on their own convictions. Lay people who are not patients or patient activists have also to rely on their convictions. Convictions are settled beliefs (Brown, 1993). They may be based on 'ordinary' knowledge or on informed or expert knowledge (Schutz, 1964). 'Ordinary' people tend to hold unclarified views based on vague knowledge; experts to hold reasoned and articulated views (Schutz, 1964). But experts and ordinary people can hold the same conviction about something, for or against capital punishment, say, for the same or for different reasons. Convictions are based on strong feelings and give energy to action. They also lead to conflict and schism.

Schisms are divisions that engender and reflect mutual hostility, splits between people who were, or who might be expected to be, unified (Little et al, 1936; Brown, 1993). They are common in recognised emancipation movements (Goodwin et al, 2001). In the women's movement, there are at least nine different sets of ideas and beliefs (Tong, 1997). The black civil rights movement in Chicago has been torn by strife (Waite, 2001). Underlying some of the conflicts and schisms are probably issues about who should speak for (represent) the oppressed social group, as well as about what they should say.

Patient activists, meeting each other for the first time or starting to work together, can feel immediate rapport or immediate antipathy. Patient groups can have difficulties working with each other, difficulties sometimes so great as to prevent collaboration. Groups and individuals readily see each other as "too way out" and "rocking the boat" or as "too cosy with health professionals" and "too supine" towards them (Williamson, 2008a). "She's a menace", "he's hopeless", sum up each other. However evident and bitter the conflicts, though, the sets of convictions, the positions, behind them are often obscure.

A major source of antipathy and conflict is, I think, the radical–conservative dimension postulated by Borkman as running across patient groups (Chapter Three; Borkman, 1997). People may have a general propensity to react conservatively or radically to specific situations; different reactions can be seen in healthcare professionals and in lay people as well as in patient groups and patient activists (Chapter Nine). In this chapter, I look at evidence for the existence of a radical–conservative dimension in groups charged with representing (speaking for) the interests of patients. First, I revisit some research I did in the early 1980s, then I consider how its findings compare with what we can observe today.

Background: lay people in health service governance bodies

Lay people have been members of health service management or governance bodies in the UK since laymen founded non-religious hospitals in the 18th century (Abel-Smith, 1964). This tradition continued when the NHS took over the hospitals in 1948. Governments assumed that lay members (reputable citizens and local authority councillors) could protect the interests of patients, as part of their work of governance. However, in a series of inquiries into hospital scandals, starting in the late 1960s and continuing intermittently ever since, lay members have been criticised for failing to notice lamentable standards of care ('no reasonably observant and caring person would have been satisfied with conditions' in Normansfield Hospital); or to have disregarded them; or to have had 'unenlightened attitudes towards patients' (Ely Hospital); or to have deferred to the expertise or the views of doctors in the hospitals; or to have thought that they must not criticise anything that could be termed 'clinical' or a matter of 'clinical judgement' (DHSS, 1969; DHSS, 1971; DHSS, 1972; DHSS, 1974a; DHSS, 1978). Some lay members refused even to listen to criticisms of care.

◊◊ When, in the early 1970s, I telephoned the chair of a hospital management committee [NHS governance body] to ask if I could see her to discuss my concerns about the care of mentally handicapped (learning disabled) children in one of her hospitals, she refused, saying that she would "follow [the consultant in mental handicap] to the ends of the earth". ◊◊

Revelations that lay members of governance bodies could not or did not protect patients' interests led policy makers to believe that the representation of patients' interests should be separated from the managerial responsibilities of governance (Klein and Lewis, 1976; Harrison and McDonald, 2008). In 1974 the government split governance from representation by setting up community health councils (CHCs) to represent patients' and the community's interests to local health service management or governance bodies (Klein and Lewis, 1976). Every health district, the unit of administration based on the population served by a district general hospital, had a CHC, in England and Wales, and in Scotland, a local health board (Department of Health and Social Security, 1974b). CHCs had between 18 and 30 unpaid lay members and a paid secretary. The lay members were a mix of local authority councillors and members of local patient or health-related voluntary groups and organisations, with a few other miscellaneous lay people. Members of patient pressure groups, support groups for patients or for local hospitals, service-providing groups, and community and race relations groups were eligible for appointment: the exact composition at any time depended on local circumstances and the turn-over of members. The government assigned CHCs various duties, one of which was 'to keep under review the operation of the health services in its district and make recommendations for the improvement of such service or otherwise advise any relevant Area Health Authority [the local NHS governance body] upon such matters relating to the operation of the health service within its district as the Council thinks fit' (Statutory Instrument 1973 No. 2217). CHCs were directed to assess standards of care, such as visiting arrangements for hospital patients, and had a statutory right to visit health service premises for this purpose (Statutory Instrument 1973 No. 2217).

Community Health Councils

From CHCs' earliest days, commentators remarked on the variability of CHCs' performance and on the propensity of their members to engage in conflicts with each other or with their CHC secretary (chief officer) (Hallas, 1976; Cang, 1978; Farrell and Levitt, 1980).

◊◊ '[In some CHCs] the debate had one leaning forward so as not to miss any of the sarcastic remarks and the cutting-edged comments flying about.' (Hallas, 1976, p 3) ◊◊

When members and secretaries from different CHCs met, they sometimes showed disdain for each other (Williamson, 1983). One cause of conflict was surmised by Stephen Cang in 1978, listening to CHC members and secretaries talking. He put forward an hypothesis that CHC members located themselves on a continuum between two incompatible 'choices', A and B, 'identification with people and groups in the community who needed health services and wanted to see improvements in them', and 'identification with the NHS', that is, with providers, staff and management (Cang, 1978). But Cang said that the principles that lay under those choices remained obscure (Cang, 1978).

As a member of Northallerton CHC, North Yorkshire, from 1974 to 1976, I had noticed that my colleagues took the side of staff, not of patients, when there was a conflict of interests over standards of care. Colleagues seemed more concerned with staff's welfare than with that of patients (Williamson, 1983). CHCs' annual reports also showed that CHCs regularly took different positions on this point, some apparently taking the side of patients, others that of staff.

Research

As part of research into what CHCs were doing about standards of care, I found 10 pairs of opposite positions in the annual reports for 1976/77 and 1977/ 78 of a random sample of 45 out of 203 CHCs in England. To see if there were any patterns in what seemed meaningless data, I did a principal component analysis of these data (Williamson, 1983). Principal component analysis is a mathematical way of handling data that may be too numerous or too confusing to handle in their original form and whose relations in those data may be entirely obscure

(Marriott, 1974). The analysis explores the mathematical nature and number of latent variables under those data, combining them into a set of new variables, the principal components (Marriott, 1974). These new variables are real in a mathematical sense. But what they mean in words has to be inferred inductively by comparing them with other data. The Appendix gives a fuller account of the method.

The first principal component gave a score to each CHC and accounted for most of the variation in the data and so was the most important. It was a bipolar continuous variable with high positive scores at one end of the continuum and high negative scores at the other, and medium and low scores in the middle. The distribution of CHCs' scores is shown in Figure A.1 in the Appendix. The pairs of incompatible or opposite positions that were used in the analysis, and their numerical scores that showed their relative weighting or influence on the first principal component, are shown in Table 8.1.

Looking at the rank order of the weightings of the incompatible positions led me to think that the first principal component was a measure of whether CHCs supported patients' interests both when they coincided and when they conflicted with those of staff, or supported patients' interests only when they coincided with those of staff. In Alford's terms, some CHCs supported dominant interests; others supported patients' repressed interests even when they conflicted with dominant interests. Alford said that most people support dominant interests; that is largely how dominant interests maintain their dominance (Alford, 1975). Fortunately for my interpretation of what the first principal component meant, there were more CHCs whose scores indicated that they predominantly supported dominant interests, 29, than there were CHCs who predominantly supported repressed interests, 16 (see Figure A.1 in the Appendix).

Another way of expressing this is to use the terms radical and conservative. A few CHCs, with high scores at one end of the continuum, were strongly radical, opposing some of the standards of care in place in their health district, the status quo. A few CHCs, with high scores at the other end of the continuum were strongly conservative, supporting local professionals' standards of care. Most had scores in between, as shown in Figure A.1 in the Appendix, and so were moderately to weakly radical or moderately to weakly conservative. The 'choices' that Borkman and Cang said that people made were choices that they made from conviction, not necessarily from conscious ideological or political positions. Members' convictions led to conflicts when they were incompatible with other members' convictions.

The rank order of the weightings was also significant (see Table 8.1). The higher the score for each pair of incompatible positions, the more important they were as contributing to the radical–conservative dimension of the CHCs. Members' convictions (and the internal dynamics within each CHC that favoured some convictions rather than others, if they conflicted) mattered. The five most important pairs of incompatible positions were: mode of representation; alignment with staff or alignment with patients; approval or disapproval of health education; whether to speak for the community's views to the NHS or to act as a broker between the community and the NHS; and training for CHC members valued or not valued.

Table 8.1: The loading on the first principal component of ten pairs of community health councils' incompatible positions

Position on	Conservative	Radical	Loading on the first principal component
Representation	do not consult with patients or with the community	pro-active consultation	5.25
Staff	praise staff, no criticism	appraise staff, including criticism	4.59
Health education	take part	do not take part	4.56
Aim	to represent NHS to the community and to act as mediator	to represent patients and the community to the NHS	4.09
Training for CHC members	not valued	valued	3.83
Management	good relationship, collaborative	collaborative but some criticisms	3.03
Patients' complaints	little attention	much attention	2.77
Location of office	on hospital premises	in high street	2.41
Membership of ACHCEW	not joined	joined	2.21
Members' voluntary organisations named	named	not named	−1.67

1. Mode of representation (weighting on first principal component, 5.25)

Radical CHCs took the representation of patients' and the community's interests to management to entail active consultation with patient and community groups and/or research into the views and needs of such groups. Conservative CHCs made no mention of active consultation or of research, relying on CHC members' views instead.

This variable, mode of representation, that is, this conflict over convictions about what representation was, weighed more heavily than any other on the radical–conservative dimension. It had (and still has) profound implications.

Radical CHCs gave 'voice' to patients, a crucial step in lifting repression from their interests (Chapter Two). All patient groups stress the importance of consulting patients and paying attention to their views (Baggott et al, 2005). Radical, knowledgeable CHCs also studied standards of care published by the Department of Health and Social Security, professional bodies and patient groups (Williamson, 1983). The link between knowledge and radicalness is close (see Conclusions at the end of this chapter).

Conservative CHCs relied mainly on their members' personal knowledge and common sense. Personal knowledge is limited and common sense in healthcare reflects common, that is, dominant, views and values. 'Lay' knowledge on its own will tend to support dominant interests (Hogg and Williamson, 2001). People with only lay knowledge of healthcare will seldom be in touch with patients' or patient groups' views (Davies, 2001).

Incompatible convictions about what is meant by 'representation' are familiar to political scientists (Pitkin, 1967). Democratic representation through elected representatives like local authority councillors and Members of Parliament; or representation through directly consulting populations and groups; or representation through the expertise of individuals and groups who have studied the views and interests of various categories of people, are some of the meanings that 'representation' can have (Pitkin, 1967).

Local authority councillors, particularly, tend to see their own views as standing in for the views and interests of the people for whom they speak (Dearlove, 1973). Local authority councillors are elected on party political manifestos. (They are not elected on healthcare political manifestos, since there are no such manifestos in the UK.) As a matter of democratic principle, councillors rely on general and common-sense knowledge (Dearlove, 1973). They tend to value the 'general will' of the whole community and think that the wishes of specialist groups will conflict with the general will (Newton, 1976). The general will tends to support dominant interests (Alford, 1975). So, like other lay and 'ordinary' people, councillors will tend to support the status quo and the repression of patients' interests, when those interests conflict with those of dominant interest holders.

Conservative CHCs were statistically significantly more likely than radical CHCs to have more than one-third members who were local authority councillors. Conservative CHCs were also more likely to contain members of leagues of hospital friends. Radical CHCs were more likely than conservative CHCs to contain members of NAWCH or race relations groups. This last finding made a direct link between radical CHCs and radical patient or community groups.

2. Alignment with staff or alignment with patients (relative weighting, 4.59)

Radical CHCs' reports appraised hospital staff, criticising or praising their work in detail. They discriminated between good and poor care, high and low standards, and commented accordingly. Conservative CHCs made no criticisms, describing staff's work as 'dedicated' or 'devoted' or thanking them for it.

◊◊ '... the gentleness and courtesy of staff in their handling of psychogeriatric patients.' *Radical CHC* (a CHC whose members had spent many hours observing care on a psychogeriatric ward) ◊◊

◊◊ 'We learn all too often of thoughtless and sometimes irresponsible actions by doctors.' *Radical CHC* ◊◊

◊◊ 'Medical staff should attempt to arrive on time [at out-patient clinics] ... stockpiling of patients is inexcusable.' *Radical CHC* ◊◊

◊◊ 'We would like to express admiration and respect for all the many professions involved in patient care. Their immense concern for all their patients ... is a real inspiration to us.' *Conservative CHC* ◊◊

◊◊ '[We apologise for] our intrusion [on staff's time on CHC visits to health service premises].' *Conservative CHC* (CHCs had a statutory right and duty to visit.) ◊◊

It is seldom clear whether people align themselves with staff because they feel some kind of kinship with them (identification) or whether they do not know how to tell the difference between staff's interests and patients' interests. Distinguishing between patients' interests that conflict with those of staff and those that coincide with them is a question partly of knowledge, partly of political alignment. Supporting staff's views and interests is often the default position, that is, lay people and activists may support professional staff because they are unaware of conflicts of interest (Chapter Three). But sometimes conservative CHCs supported staff's interests when they knew that they conflicted with patients' interests.

◊ ◊ A *conservative* CHC supported staff's and the area health authority's policy that children could only visit their mothers in a maternity unit for one hour once a week, in spite of a public campaign by parents and the criticism of the restriction by the Health Service Commissioner. The Minister for Health intervened, and an experimental period of visiting by children for one hour per day was set up a year later. But it culminated in a total ban on child visitors two and a half years later, after contraction of the visiting times and the restriction of the children to day rooms had created overcrowding and given nurses the problem of controlling unruly children. The CHC supported this policy also (*Annual Reports*, 1975/76, 1976/77, 1979/80 and press coverage). ◊ ◊

By contrast:

◊ ◊ A strongly *radical* CHC discovered that a new paediatric ward sister had introduced restricted visiting by parents. CHC members promptly visited the ward, took the matter up with management, and got unrestricted visiting restored. ◊ ◊

This variable, with the second-heaviest weighting on the radical–conservative dimension, reminds us that patients who have been radicalised tend to criticise some health professionals severely (Chapter Four). Uncritical admiration of professionals' actions sustains the repression of patients' interests.

3. Approval or disapproval of health education (relative weighting, 4.56)

Health education can be seen as offering patients and the public useful information and advice. Or it can be seen as attempting to persuade (educate) patients and the public to behave in ways that accord with professional or managerial instructions and priorities. Some CHCs took no part in health education, other CHCs mentioned various projects approvingly: radical and conservative, respectively.

Conservative CHCs tended to accept health education's didacticism and chided patients for things like smoking and abuse of the health service. Radical CHCs recognised that there were problems but directed their censure towards the health service, not towards patients.

◊◊ 'The general public will have to be disabused of the belief that ambulances are in competition with other forms of transport and are available for trips to town.' *Conservative CHC* ◊◊

◊◊ 'While recognising abuse of the hospital transport schemes as well as its enormous cost we believe nevertheless that economies and exhortations to doctors to order less transport will lead to a deterioration in the health of a large number of patients and that geographical inequalities will become even greater than they are now. We believe that the state has a responsibility for providing as good health care for those living in rural areas as in towns.' *Radical CHC* ◊◊

◊◊ '... the appointments system is of the "block-booking" type whereby a number of patients are given the same time for an appointment so as to make maximum use of consultants' time and avoid unnecessary gaps. Whilst on occasions, clinics may have to be cancelled and time does not permit for patients to be notified and given advance warning, there are a number of patients who for their part, fail to keep an appointment without notifying the hospital and so waste the clinicians' time.' *Conservative CHC* ◊◊

This pair of positions prompts the question, whose side were some of these CHCs on?

Health education (and its offspring, self-care) is still controversial because of its coercive aspects (Steinbrook, 2006).

4. Training for CHC members valued or not valued (relative weighting, 3.83)

Radical CHCs said that they valued training for members or listed the conferences and seminars that their members had attended. Conservative CHCs said they did not value training or listed few or no conferences.

> ◊◊ 'Members' commitments include participating in seminars, attending conferences, lectures, study groups ... studying various documents and papers in preparation for meetings.' *Radical CHC* ◊◊

> ◊◊ 'If we so wished, members could be attending conferences on one subject or another at very frequent intervals ... they are expensive and time-consuming events and useless to anyone but the individual concerned unless there is proper feed-back.' *Conservative CHC* ◊◊

That training was neither necessary nor desirable was explicitly linked to 'lay' status by some CHC members.

> ◊◊ "One should be acting as an everyday person and training would remove this." (Local authority councillor member, interview, 1980) ◊◊

These four variables were important for the radical–conservative dimension. They or their descendants are still relevant today. (I omit one CHC variable – aim – that has little relevance today.)

Conflict and stress in CHCs

Because it was possible to tell from CHCs' scores for the first principal component whether a CHC was radical or conservative, I could match what their members said about their experiences in their CHCs to their CHCs' conservatism or radicalness. In essence, radical members in radical CHCs were happy. In conservative CHCs, radical members were unhappy, unable to achieve as much as they would like for standards of care and sometimes feeling isolated and stressed.

◊◊ "Any subject [I raise] is welcomed as long as it's seriously talked about … a particularly good CHC membership, intelligent people." *Radical member in radical CHC* ◊◊

◊◊ "Though I only raise issues [of standards of care] if making proposals that would end in action, members say 'good, what shall we do with it?'" *Radical member in radical CHC* ◊◊

◊◊ "There are lots of issues I'd like to raise but my battling spirit is lost." *Radical member in conservative CHC* ◊◊

◊◊ "When I try to get something done, [the other members] feel that the 'emotional involvement' of women is too much, they say they have no rational judgement of what goes on." *Radical member in conservative CHC* ◊◊

◊◊ "I don't seem to get it over … they don't grasp … issues of 'psychological comfort', only concrete ones like a lavatory chain which doesn't pull." *Radical member in conservative CHC* ◊◊

Vignette of two CHCs

All CHCs did useful work. But strongly radical and strongly conservative CHCs differed markedly from each other.

◊◊ A strongly conservative CHC, Calderdale, in 1980/81, was concerned with the provision of a new laundry; the building of a new mental handicap hospital; more toilet accommodation in a ward; a supervised play area in a health centre; improvements to a pram shelter at a clinic; and more sessions at another clinic. (*Calderdale CHC Annual Report for 1980/81*). These were improvements that would benefit patients and staff, giving staff pleasanter working environments, better facilities, more posts. (Building a new mental handicap hospital was possibly outmoded, though.) ◊◊

◊◊ A strongly radical CHC, Central Birmingham, in 1978/79, wished to see the appointment of a consultant paediatric ophthalmologist; the provision of a covered way between ward and theatre at a children's hospital; rubella vaccination; a circumcision service for Muslim babies; the setting up of a district handicap team; and a hostel for mentally handicapped people

(*Central Birmingham CHC Annual Report for 1978/79*). So this CHC, too, wanted improvements that would benefit patients and staff, giving staff pleasanter working environments, more posts, more varied work. ◊◊

Central Birmingham CHC, in addition, criticised clinical and managerial decisions. It made public a decision of ophthalmologists to treat a small number of patients by sophisticated and time-consuming techniques in partial preference to a larger number of patients who needed only simple operations. It 'was shocked to find that in Birmingham the kind of psychiatric treatment you get depends on where you live' and suggested steps to remedy this. It discovered that women's chances of admission to a local obstetric 'centre of excellence' were positively related to their social class, in spite of the known inverse relationship between class and perinatal mortality (*Central Birmingham CHC Annual Report for 1978/79*). Table 8.2 emphasises these points: one quarter of the diagram is empty.

Table 8.2: A radical and a conservative community health council

CHC requests provision of facilities or services	CHC criticises doctors' decisions, how services are provided or delivered
Central Birmingham, radical	
consultant paediatric ophthalmologist	ophthalmologists' decision to do one kind of procedure rather than another
covered way between ward and theatre	psychiatric services are by postcode
circumcision service	lower social classes get worse obstetric care
rubella vaccination	
district handicap team	
hostel for people with mental handicap	
Calderdale, conservative	
new laundry	
new mental handicap hospital	
toilet accommodation on ward	
supervised play area	
pram shelter	
provide more clinic sessions	

Relevance to today: radical and conservative patient groups and patient activists

This CHC research gave evidence, independent of Borkman's paper 15 years later, for the existence of a radical–conservative dimension that cuts across not just patient groups, but also lay people and patient activists who are expected to represent the interests of patients. Radicalness and conservatism are most easily detected in groups or individuals that are either strongly radical or strongly conservative. Radicalness and conservatism are also more easily detected in groups than in individuals, perhaps because groups, in reports or other publications, express their positions on several issues, individuals usually on only one or two at a time.

Today's patient groups can be radical or conservative or in between (Chapter Three). Today's radical patient groups' publications are likely to contain criticisms of the service and of policies, practices and standards, often through patients' accounts of their experiences. Articles, papers and reviews are likely to raise and discuss issues in detail. Strongly conservative groups' publications seldom contain criticisms of the service, either in general or of particular clinical or managerial arrangements. Yet no service is faultless, from patients', or from any other, perspective. Staying silent on a topic or issue expresses a position on it. The dog that didn't bark in the night, in the Sherlock Holmes story 'Silver Blaze', took the position that the person prowling round in the dark was a friend, not a stranger (Conan Doyle, 1928).

◊◊ In 2008, the International Glaucoma Association's journal, *iga News,* gave members information in articles by ophthalmologists on topics like surgery in the treatment of glaucoma; why field tests are important; and what sorts of apparatus are used for measuring pressures in the eyes. Ophthalmologists also answered questions sent in by members and explained problems and risks in treatments. The journal included reports on fundraising, support groups and increasing the public's awareness of glaucoma. It had no criticisms of the services by ophthalmologists or by patients (*iga News*, 2008, Spring, Summer, Autumn). *Conservative patient organisation* ◊◊

◊◊ In 2008, the Association for Improvements in the Maternity Services' journal, *AIMS Journal*, had articles on cultural perspectives on mothering; women's regrets about not having been assertive enough when in labour; post-traumatic stress disorder caused by distressing experiences of childbirth; hospitals' conflicting policies on breast feeding; 'women as obstetric fashion victims' (*AIMS Journal* 2008, vol 20, nos 1–4). *Radical patient group* ◊◊

It would be fairly easy to apply a principal component analysis to a sample of patient groups' positions, taken perhaps from their annual reports or journals. Some divisive issues and incompatible positions will have disappeared or changed, but probably not all, and others will have emerged. Positions that might turn out to be associated with conservatism include: having paid staff; having a majority of health professionals on the group's governance body; accepting money from pharmaceutical companies; praising healthcare professionals and current treatments; playing down the risks of treatments; and emphasising patients' responsibilities for keeping appointments and for taking their medication. Positions that might turn out to be associated with radicalness include: being purely a voluntary (unpaid) group; having no or few health professionals on the governance body; rejecting money from pharmaceutical companies; praising some healthcare professionals but criticising others; stressing the risks of some treatments; giving patients' accounts of their poor care; and emphasising patients' rights. These are all currently controversial issues among patient groups and patient activists.

Today's conservative patient activists are more likely to hold repressive views than emancipating views; today's radical activists more likely to hold emancipating ideas, those that support the autonomy of patients, individually and collectively. Conservative activists' views on issues that are controversial within the medical profession are more likely to accord with those of conservative doctors, radical activists' views with those of radical doctors (Chapter Nine). Radical doctors are more likely than conservative doctors to favour telling patients about treatments that their primary healthcare trust will not pay for; that they are being put at risk by delays in radiotherapy; and so on (Chapters Two and Seven). So for some issues, conservative patient activists and professionals form one camp and radical activists and professionals another, looking at each other across a chasm.

Today's controversies and conflicts

In today's controversies in healthcare, we can still pick up descendants of the four most controversial issues for CHCs in the late 1970s and early 1980s:

1. Mode of representation

CHCs have gone. They were abolished by the government in 2003 (Gerrard, 2006; Hogg, 2009). But ambiguities and tensions around representation continue to flourish, as the government, official and professional bodies appoint lay people and patients to advisory and policy-making groups.

The issue of who can legitimately speak for patients' interests is probably even more controversial now than it was 20 years ago. The implications of conflicting views of representation are perhaps more apparent. Patients are more clearly differentiated into patients, patient-group members and patient representatives/advocates (Chapter Seven). Lumping together the public, lay people, non-activist patients and patient activists, instead of seeking views from each category by appropriate methods, supports dominant interests. So does seeking the views of only one or a few categories of people.

At the same time, people making appointments have perhaps begun to recognise radicalness and conservatism, though they probably seldom put that into words. Some radical patient activists believe that their applications for memberships of official bodies were rejected because they were too knowledgeable about the group's task, and therefore likely to be thought too radical.

◊◊ "I shall remain a guerrilla on the outside," said an activist who was not appointed to the governance body of a regulatory authority, though she was exceptionally well qualified, having researched regulation in healthcare (personal communication, 2001). ◊◊

◊◊ A radical activist was asked at interview for another regulatory body whether poachers could turn into gamekeepers. She was not appointed (personal communication, 2006). ◊◊

As radicalness and conservatism become easier to identify, some official bodies will be tempted to appoint only conservative activists. But other appointing bodies have valued, and will continue to value, radical activists.

2. Alignment with staff or alignment with patients

The belief that lay people (people without a health professional qualification) are aligned with patients and can speak for their interests dies hard (Hogg and Williamson, 2001). Even when representation is separated from management and governance, lay people tend to side with health professionals or with corporate rationalisers. They seem to feel more sympathy for staff and for managers than for patients. Or they see certain practices and standards as legitimate that (radical) patient activists would see as coercive (Chapter Three). Or they do not know how to judge standards of care (Williamson, 1987). Or they, like some patients, may excuse poor care or low standards because they believe that staff are doing their best (Edwards et al, 2004). Unconscious feelings and fantasies are likely to be important, too, for lay people (and patient activists) can easily imagine themselves as vulnerable patients (Chapter Nine). We all need to trust that professionals will treat us well, should we need their help. Emotionally, it is more comfortable to support professionals and their interests than to oppose them. Intellectually and politically, it is easier to support dominant interest holders than to oppose them or what they do (Chapter Three). Most lay people and many patients do support those interests; that is how dominant interests retain their dominance (Alford, 1975).

These points are usually obscured by the health service's noble rhetoric and ignoble cant. Besides, everyone who supports patients' interests that are compatible with dominant interests can believe that they act in patients' interests. In a limited but true sense, they do.

Alignment with staff or with corporate rationalisers, expressed as alignment with dominant interests (Chapter Two), does not mean that those who support dominant interests feel hostility or indifference towards patients. Similarly, alignment with patients, better expressed as alignment with repressed interests, does not mean hostility towards health professionals, although professionals and radical activists can feel antagonism towards each other, if their views over sensitive issues conflict (Chapter Nine).

Like CHCs before them, groups of mixed lay people, conservative and radical activists can feel stress if there are mismatches between members.

◊◊ "We are here to support doctors, not to criticise them," said the chair of a patient liaison group of a medical royal college, causing dismay to the radical members present at a meeting (radical member, personal communication, 2007). ◊◊

◊◊ During a discussion in a patient liaison group of standards of care in a medical royal college, a confident, articulate lay member was quick to endorse whatever the medical members said. The radical patient activist members opposed his views. He later resigned (personal observation, 2000). ◊◊

3. Approval or disapproval of health education

The disapproval of patients who fail to conform to dominant interest holders' interests and prescriptions for the ways in which patients should behave that was evident in the sample of CHCs 30 years ago, and was then associated with conservatism, is still salient today.

> ◊◊ An independent advocate for quality in research and healthcare wrote about whether patients should be allowed to buy unlicensed drugs undergoing clinical trials and not provided by their primary healthcare trust as part of NHS treatment.'This new class of "active" patient, wealthy enough to purchase expensive ... drugs such as Herceptin (trastuzumab), could add a new, unbalancing component to shared decision making, by rendering clinicians scarcely more than technicians.The effect on the research process would do a disservice to fellow patients with breast cancer and be disruptive to equitable and evidence based provision of health care ... The conduct and quality of research globally would ... be diminished. (Thornton, 2002, p 110). ◊◊

> ◊◊ The chair of a patient liaison group wrote: '[I] particularly enjoyed the short-tempered reaction of the nightshift accident and emergency doctor to the inappropriate and time-wasting queries from serial hypochondriacs' (Cropper, 2008, p 310). ◊◊

These extracts deal with undoubted problems for researchers, clinicians and desperate patients. But their tone towards patients is like that of some conservative CHCs. Like them, they are inclined to attribute the problems solely to patients rather than to shortages of money, staff, time, skill or imagination in the health service.They seem to frown on actions by patients that have not been legitimated by a higher authority. In this, they are like the punitive doctors in the section on Equity in Chapter Seven.

This variable could be confused with *alignment with staff versus alignment with patients*, 2 above, and probably overlaps with it. In the CHC sample, the two together added up to the largest proportion of the variance between radical and conservative CHCs, almost more than twice as much as the highest-loading variable, mode of representation (mode of representation, 5.25, alignment with staff or patients, 4.59, participation or not in health education, 4.56). Combining them into a single variable would simplify things, provided we remember that what looks like a simple variable has complex bases in knowledge, feelings and political alignments.

4. Training for members valued or not valued

The issues of lay knowledge versus professional knowledge, naiveté versus expertise, generalism versus specialism, experience versus academic study, are salient today. (These are continuous variables, but people often see them as dichotomies.) What sorts of training and knowledge might be relevant for what sorts of lay people, patients and patient activists who are appointed or expected to represent lay or patients' interests; who could provide it; who would pay for it, are even more pressing issues than they were in the days of CHCs. CHCs could arrange training, get documents and other resources for their members. Resources for patient activists are now more haphazard.

◊◊ The patient activist members of a working party at the MHRA (Chapter Seven) asked to view a BBC *Panorama* programme that threw doubt on the regulation of the controversial drug seroxat (paroxetine). The request was refused. ◊◊

◊◊ The College of Health, a national patient organisation, now defunct, said that advanced training would distance activists from 'ordinary' patients, when I asked it about training in the 1990s. ◊◊

This view, whether expressed or not, probably underlies a general reluctance to offer or fund advanced education or training for activists or to provide resources for them to meet their own needs for knowledge and for communication with each other (Chapter Two). These lacks support the status quo and dominant interests.

Conclusions

CHCs were ideal material for research, being uniform in some ways but diverse in others. In the CHC sample, representation through consultation and research; alignment with patients; scepticism about health education; and setting a high value on training, were associated with radicalness. Representation through personal knowledge; alignment with professional staff; approval of health education; and setting a low value on training were associated with conservatism. All these concepts are analytically distinct. But in practice they can be hard to separate.

Knowledge and radicalness are especially closely linked to each other. It can be difficult to tell the difference between someone with a radical approach or outlook and someone who knows enough to be able to challenge or oppose what is being said by professionals (Beverley Beech, radical patient activist, personal communication, 2007; Chapter Five). But although knowing enough is a necessary condition for challenging dominant interest holders, it is not a sufficient one. Some conservative patient activists are highly knowledgeable. Telling knowledgeable conservative and radical activists apart depends on judging whether they use their knowledge for restrictive or for emancipatory purposes, for challenging trivial or for challenging fundamental aspects of standards, research protocols and proposals for change. The views of individual radical and conservative patient activists can, in any case, overlap, just as CHCs' convictions did. Again, whether a view is radical or conservative depends on when it is expressed in relation to the history of an issue (Chapter Three). The intuitive feelings of radical and conservative activists about each other remain important markers.

Table 8.3: Three ways of expressing radical and conservative alignments

1	Alignment with repressed interest holders	Alignment with dominant interest holders
2	Support for patients' interests when they conflict as well as when they coincide with professionals' interests	Support of patients' interests only when they coincide with professionals' interests
3	Radical	Conservative

Table 8.3 puts together three ways of expressing radical and conservative alignments.

Various questions arise from the considerations in this chapter.

* Do radicalness and conservatism, with their four supporting sets of positions, constitute a schism within the patient movement? Do they constitute two coherent and consistent schools of thought, even though those schools of thought are unarticulated, and even though individuals and groups can hold mixed convictions? I think the answer is yes.

- Are there other important variables, other sets of incompatible positions, that reflect and contribute to this schism? Almost certainly, yes.

- Are there other important hidden variables that cause different schisms? I don't know, but I suspect that the answer is yes.

- Is all this important? Yes, because clarity about what different individuals and groups, both conservative and radical, can contribute to policies and standards in healthcare is essential, if patients' interests are to be protected and if the quality of healthcare is to be raised. Yes, because of the connection between radicalness and emancipation (Chapter Three).

NINE

Allies and antagonists

We need to work with people who do not doubt our good intentions,
but are prepared to tell us things that others will not.

(Helen Williams, pathologist, 2003, p 33)

Introduction

Doctors can be radical patient activism's best friends or worst enemies. This chapter looks at radical doctors and at conservative doctors, the allies and antagonists of the title. Most doctors are conservative to varying degrees, accepting the status quo; they tend to be antagonistic towards radical patient activism. A minority of doctors are radical, questioning the status quo; they tend to support radical patient activists' ideas and definitions of higher standards. These differences are little recognised, either in general or when doctors and patient activists work together to formulate new standards of care. Three examples are drawn on to explore some of the difficulties of this work, as well as its potential for articulating standards that meet the perspectives, purposes and interests of both doctors and patient activists.

Conservative and radical doctors

Conservative doctors tend to support the status quo, the standards in place at a given time, and radical doctors tend to question or oppose some of them. Conservative doctors tend to limit the freedom and responsibility of patients to choose how to act and radical doctors tend to support or promote those freedoms and responsibilities.

◊◊ '... doctors do actually care more about healthcare and more about their patients than anyone else does ... [m]ore even than patients themselves, who are often not in the best position, mentally or physically, to make the best judgement, no matter how much "information" they are deluged with. Doctors care mainly because that's what motivates us, partly because our enormous responsibilities mean that we have to ...'. (Lee, 2005, p 59) *Conservative* ◊◊

◊ ◊ 'We are happy to acknowledge that patients have the right to greater autonomy but ask them to acknowledge our professional right to avoid exposing them to what we consider unnecessary risks. We undertake to fulfil our responsibility of care towards them but ask in return that they act responsibly to help us keep them as safe as possible … [In offering patients information that makes them more powerful, I hope for] subtle and enlightened shifts towards equality of both power and responsibility in the innumerable human encounters that take place between anaesthetists and patients every day.' (Smith, 2003, p 411) *Radical* ◊ ◊

The first is repressive, the second liberating or emancipatory.

Allies: radical doctors

… my views on sensitive issues [were] accepted and used in national guidelines … [by the Royal College of Pathologists].

(Mitzi Blennerhasset, radical patient activist, 2008, p 184)

Some doctors and other professionals have supported the ideas and work of (radical) patient groups since the late 1950s (Williamson, 1992; Hogg, 1999). Such supporters can be called radical because, in supporting radical views, they too challenge the status quo, the dominant values, policies, practices and standards of care of their own profession. They are akin to the Britons who sought to end Britain's part in the slave trade in the 18th and 19th centuries. They are akin, too, to the men of goodwill who support the women's movement (Tong, 1997). Like them, they excite praise from some of their peers and odium from others. Like them, they lead their peers towards accepting ideas that, as they become widely accepted, change from being radical to being conservative. Gaining dominant power holders' support for specific proposals or changes is essential for radical patient activism, just as gaining powerful men's support for specific changes to customary ways of doing things is essential for the women's and other emancipation movements.

There is no easy, objective way of identifying doctors who are radical in their approach to standards of care. Radical patient activists can recognise radical doctors intuitively, that is, without conscious analysis, through those doctors' responses to them, just as they recognise kindred spirits among other activists (Chapter Eight). Radical doctors understand more quickly what radical patient activists say; do not get upset, defensive or aggressive when conflicts of view emerge; seem less dependent on rules and less fearful of going outside them; accept and, if they are in a position to, implement high standards of care as patient activists define them (conversations and interviews with radical patient activists, 2007, 2008).

Like patient activists, radical doctors show a range of degrees of radicalness, whose expression is partly influenced by the reactions they evoke from their peers. Dr Andrew Smith suggested that radical doctors can be imagined as lying on a line of continuous variation from the latently radical, through the overtly radical, to the intolerably radical (personal communication, 2008). I am greatly indebted to him for telling me his ideas and for distinguishing three grades of radical doctor on the continuum.

1. **Latent radicals** may be unaware of their radical tendencies; or keep them hidden; or not act on them. They do not usually oppose others' radical ideas and their radicalness can sometimes be mobilised in a committee or group, if an issue is presented skilfully or if shared feelings about an issue develop within the group.

2. **Overt radicals** take openly radical positions on some issues but seldom press them directly against strong opposition. They may, however, seek ways round issues or opponents in order to gain the same ends.

3. **Intolerable radicals** raise "too many" radical issues "too far" for their peers. (They are like the "way out" or "boat-rocking" radical patient activists of Chapter Eight.) Or they introduce practices into their own clinical work that deviate so far from their colleagues' policies, practices and standards that those colleagues cannot tolerate them and act against the deviant doctor.

> ◊◊ An anaesthetist who allowed, even welcomed, fathers into theatre to see the births of their babies by planned caesarean section under general anaesthetic, before this began to be tolerated elsewhere (Chapter Six), seems to have been punished by failing to achieve the career that his competence should have guaranteed (Andrew Smith, personal communication, 2008). ◊◊

This continuous series of variations or gradations can be thought of as closely akin to the radical component of the bipolar continuous variable of Chapter Eight. It is important theoretically and pragmatically. *Intolerable radicals* can be seen as pioneers who raise new issues in matters hitherto taken for granted or who show the feasibility of radical new practices or standards. These new ideas provoke opposition at first; but they may gradually become acceptable to overt and to latent radicals. Or they may not. *Overt radicals* can also be seen as pioneers when they raise new issues and articulate new, higher standards. Their greater personal acceptability to their peers makes those peers more likely to accept their ideas. *Latent radicals* go with the flow. These shades of radicalness make it easier for radical ideas to be accepted by a specialty or profession. Given that conservative doctors are in a majority, the prospects for progressive changes to standards would be bleak without these shades of radicalness and the possibility of shifts between them.

The radicalisation of doctors

Radical doctors are, by definition and by observation, a minority of the medical profession. Why some members of a subordinate, oppressed group become radicalised is easy to understand (Chapter Four). Why some members of a dominant group become radicalised is less easy to understand. Here I put forward some tentative points, based on what two well-known radical doctors, a GP and an obstetrician, have written, and on what five radical doctors, two anaesthetists, one GP, one oncologist and one pathologist, said when I interviewed them in 2008. (I knew four in their medical royal colleges, a fifth in a national patient organisation.)

Patients usually become radicalised through an intense personal experience of harm to the self, when physical or psychological harm is combined with an affront to moral agency (Chapter Four). Doctors seem to become radicalised through observing harms caused to patients by the medical profession's accustomed ways of doing things, its standards of care. The harms may be either physical or threats to the patient's moral agency. If the doctor is a medical student or a junior doctor, the actions that lead to the harms are usually taken or directed by more senior doctors. If the doctor is in autonomous practice, as a principal in general practice or as a hospital consultant, he or she may come to feel responsible for those harms.

> ◊◊ Dr (now Sir) Donald Irvine, a GP in his early practice in the 1960s, came to think that withholding from patients the knowledge that they had a serious disease like cancer, as was standard practice, was dishonest (Irvine, 2003). He changed his practice, giving patients 'more responsibility and freedom in deciding on their care' (Irvine, 2003, p 14). ◊◊

◊ ◊ Dr Wendy Savage, an obstetrician, was told by one patient that her overbearing attitude and her overriding of her [the patient's] wishes by giving her a pethidine injection during childbirth ("I've seen far more women in labour than you have") had ruined the experience of labour for her (Savage, 1986, p 18). From her patients, her work and her own experience of motherhood, Savage came to believe that women should have control over their own fertility and labours (Savage, 1986). By the late 1970s, she came to offer the fullest information to her patients, with informed choice and shared decision making, when this was rare in maternity care (Savage, 1986). ◊◊

For some radical doctors, radicalisation develops slowly and cumulatively. The surprise and shock that can trigger patients' radicalisation seem generally to be less intense. These are answers to my question "Did any specific instance radicalise you?"

◊ ◊ Dr A, when a medical student, saw that hospital staff withheld from her mother the knowledge that she had untreatable cancer and would soon die. She gradually began to see that there could be valid perspectives other than the medical one. ◊◊

◊ ◊ Dr B thought it odd to wheel in a patient in front of 200 medical students like himself in a lecture theatre, and wondered what the patient thought. ◊◊

◊ ◊ Dr C recalled three incidents:

1. In order to get a job, a West Indian woman had said she was 73, not her real age, 75. It was the hospital's policy not to resuscitate anyone 75 or over but when this woman collapsed, she was successfully resuscitated. But for her chance lie, she would not have been. Dr C felt angry about the policy, and noticed that her colleagues did not have the same reaction.

2. A man stubbed his toe on the pavement outside a hospital and went in to the Accident and Emergency Department. That started a train of treatments and iatrogenic injuries that ended with his lying in agony in a hospital bed, taking warfarin for a deep vein thrombosis. That made Dr C think "perhaps we [doctors] weren't all we were cracked up to be".

3. A patient died on the operating table, in spite of all the doctors involved in his care having looked at the notes made when he first came into hospital. It then became clear that he had had pre-existing heart disease, missed because no one had listened to what he had said, paying attention only to the notes. ◊◊

◊◊ Dr D could not recall any specific incident. ◊◊

◊◊ Dr E saw that things were wrong for patients in her clinical department of her hospital but could not change them: inhumanity seemed to be an aspect of medicine. ◊◊

Radical doctors and radical patient activists differ from each other in their power to take action. Autonomous professionals can sometimes change their own practice and that of staff junior to them. Patient activists can only bring about change through persuading professionals or corporate rationalisers, or both, to act. In spite of this advantage, radical doctors probably need as much courage and determination to go against the values, behaviours and interests of their profession as patient activists need to oppose some of its policies, practices and standards from outside it. Dr Irvine came to feel that he had to confront personally some of the 'dominant features' of the 'medical culture in which I had been brought up by the medical specialists who had taught me' and 'break free from this cultural straight-jacket' (Irvine, 2003, p 14). Dr Savage was suspended from medical practice at the instigation of her fellow obstetricians, who alleged that her practice was unsafe (Savage, 1986). This was followed by a public inquiry and her reinstatement (Savage, 1986). But although she said, 'I am not particularly a conformist, and somehow I never really felt inside the system ... I retained this scepticism', she also said, 'I did not start my medical career as a radical in the labour ward' (Savage, 1986, p 7; 1990, p 326). This sense of reluctance yet obligation is like that felt by some patients on becoming radicalised into activists (Chapter Four). But to deviate from fellow dominant interest holders' norms is probably more exacting and more painful than deviating as a repressed interest holder from the more nebulous norms of wider society.

When doctors as dominant interest holders seek to change a way of doing things that relinquishes some of their power, they threaten their profession's collective dominance. They also breach its values of mutual support and loyalty to each other. Becoming deviant by rejecting the practices and standards of fellow dominant interest holders can incur punishment.

◊◊ "I am not popular" and "My colleagues have developed antibodies to me" were rueful comments by two radical GPs, one in 1995, the other in 2008 (personal communications). ◊◊

Relations with radical patient groups

Radical professionals are important to radical patient groups. Most, probably all, such groups have working relationships with individual radical healthcare professionals. Some invite one or more onto their national committees, for example, NAWCH (paediatricians and paediatric nurses) and Breast UK (an oncologist). Or a group may work closely with a professional group, as AIMS does with the Association of Radical Midwives. This association was started in 1976 by midwives who opposed the increasing medicalisation and intervention in maternity care and wanted to revive basic midwifery skills and provide a service 'tailored more closely to [each woman's] needs, and a sympathetic attitude on the part of their professional attendants' (www.radmid.demon.co.uk). Its aims and ethos are close to those of AIMS, which publishes articles by radical midwives in its journal. Or a patient group may consult sympathetic clinicians or other healthcare-related professionals, like pharmacologists, when it needs information or advice, as APRIL does (www.april.org.uk).

Radical professionals help patient group members with technical matters and give them inside information about how their specialty thinks and works. In return, radical professionals gain esteem, emotional support and intellectual stimulus, as well as the relief of being able to talk freely without having to consider the likely reactions of their professional peers. If a professional is so intolerably radical that he or she is severely and openly punished by professional peers, patient groups can make their support public.

◊◊ AIMS and the National Childbirth Trust (NCT) (a patient group started in 1956 and at the time radical) supported Dr Savage when she was suspended from her NHS posts. They set up a campaign group with representatives of the local community health council and a local health campaign group and marched with local families through the streets of the East End of London (Savage, 1986). ◊◊

Radical doctors sometimes become famous. Drs Dermot Macarthy and David Morris, for paediatric care, and Wendy Savage and Peter Huntingford, for maternity care, in the 1960s and 1970s are examples. Though on a smaller scale, their reputations are revered like William Wilberforce's (1759–1833) for opposing the slave trade or Christabel Pankhurst's (1880–1958) for campaigning for votes for women.

Antagonists: conservative doctors

"You're not a real patient!"

(Accusation often made to patient activists by conservative doctors)

It's hard to be attacked for constructive criticism, just because we are not mindless fans [of doctors].

(Roger Goss, radical patient activist, personal communication, 2007)

We might suppose that conservative doctors would be 'naturally' antagonistic towards radical patient activism. Indeed, activists identify conservative doctors in the same way as they do radical doctors: by their reactions to them and to what they say. Doctors and other professionals whose reactions include defensiveness, avoidance or aggressiveness usually hold conservative views on issues and will seldom want to accept or change standards in progressive directions. They seem to feel safer within the status quo (Elisabeth Hartley and other radical patient activists, personal communications, 2007; 2008).

Researchers and policy analysts, however, seldom distinguish between conservatives and radicals. Because most doctors are conservative, that is, support the status quo from conviction or by default, the points that follow in the next paragraph can be assumed to apply chiefly to them. It is, however, probable that there is a continuous gradient from weakly conservative doctors through moderately conservative ones to strongly conservative ones, 'backwoods-men', in the picturesque metaphor that doctors sometimes apply to their colleagues. Latent conservatism can probably exist in some doctors who profess to be radical, just as latent radicalness can exist in some doctors who appear to be conservative. The boundary between radicalness and conservatism is not clear cut (unless mathematical criteria are used to define it, Chapter Eight). It changes over time as some radical ideas become influential and some conservative ideas decline. Individuals, too, can change their emotional, intellectual and political positions on some issues, sometimes suddenly (Chapter Ten).

The medical profession prides itself on being different from the laity and seeks to maintain its differences (Freidson, 1970b). Few doctors wish to influence their peers' or their senior colleagues' work and seldom comment on or criticise it. It is not considered clinical etiquette to do so (Armstrong and Ogden, 2006). So it is hardly surprising that, as sociologists have noted, doctors are reluctant to listen to lay ideas and lay-initiated discoveries (Brown, 2000). Lay contributions, perceptions and views are likely to be seen as conflictual (Brown, 2000). Dominant groups try to avoid conflict with members of subordinate groups because they like to believe that subordinate groups are content. 'For motives that can be entirely honourable, even idealistic, people in power often refuse to look at things that are staring them in the face' (Anon, 1998, p 39). Besides, the repression of patients' interests means that doctors are unaccustomed to hearing patients' definitions of their interests (Chapter Two), as well as unwilling (Chapter Five).

When doctors resist other people's ideas, however, they are not necessarily resisting them because the ideas are radical. Doctors tend to resist all proposed changes, unless those changes will be clearly to their advantage or will increase their power (Wagner, 1994). But some doctors' distrust of all patient groups, their suspicion of all patient advocates or representatives, pejoratively referred to as 'the usual suspects' (Hogg, 2009, p 5), and their beliefs about 'real' patients suggest an antagonism that can easily shade into hostility, irrespective of whether these patient groups and individuals are radical or conservative.

Patient groups

Hostility towards patient groups is openly expressed by some doctors. They see patient groups as selfish, seeking resources for patients like themselves and so distorting wiser, legitimate allocations; as venal, seduced by drug companies who fund their projects and publications; as fanatic, single-issue advocates, grinding their own axes; as stupid, not properly understanding healthcare; and as tedious to consult, holding up progress (Tallis, 2004; and comments heard at meetings over many years).

Double standards prevail here. Hostile doctors seldom reflect on the reasons for these shortcomings or whether, to the extent that they are shortcomings (allocations of resources are always problematic, single issues are often important), their profession is guilty of them. Some patients' organisations do accept money from pharmaceutical companies, either openly or covertly (Herxheimer, 2003). But some doctors do the same, accepting presents, meals, funding for research, funding for continuing medical education, even fees for ghost-writing reports praising a new drug (Rogers, 2007; Krumholz et al, 2009). Some doctors also hold up progress, as their own colleagues or corporate rationalisers see progress (Salter, 2004).

Patient representatives or advocates

Doctors and other healthcare professionals tend to see patient representatives or advocates as unrepresentative of patients and therefore unable to represent their interests. Confusion over the meanings of 'representative' and 'representation'; lack of recognition that patients, patient group members and patient representatives have different kinds and levels of knowledge and expertise; and lack of insight into how to judge the validity of what patient representatives say about patients' interests were discussed in Chapter Seven. This confusion is partly due to the immaturity of the patient movement and its backwardness in explaining itself or putting forward an ideology. But probably some misunderstandings are "accidentally on purpose", as children say.

In addition, doctors may feel discomfort when individual patient activists disagree with each other in meetings (Dr A, personal communication, 2004). Seeing members of subordinate social groups as all the same, inability to discern differences between them that are apparent to the groups themselves, may be characteristic of dominant interest holders. Dominant interest holders need not study repressed interest holders, whereas repressed interest holders must study dominant interest holders, if they hope to influence them (Chapter Five).

Again, double standards prevail. Doctors seem seldom to reflect on how representative of other doctors they themselves are; whether they always agree with each other; and why they respect specialised knowledge in their peers but not in patient representatives. Double standards in any sphere of life indicate inequality.

'Real' patients

Some health professionals, corporate rationalisers and commentators have a vision of the 'real' patient. 'Real' patients are patients whose knowledge of healthcare does not extend beyond their own experience of it. They are not politically or intellectually engaged with the health service. They are not trying to improve healthcare for other patients. They are the 'ordinary' patients, the majority of patients, whom clinicians see in their everyday work. Any patient who takes social action by joining a patient group or by studying healthcare beyond his or her own predicament forfeits being 'real' (Hogg and Williamson, 2001). 'Real' or naive patients are assumed to be free of vested interests (Taylor and Lupton, 1995). Their views are assumed to bubble up fresh and pure from a spring uncontaminated by the muddy grit of patient activism.

At first sight, this is an odd and confused way of looking at patients. Everyone is equally real. Knowledge is not usually regarded as contaminating. Everyone's perceptions, views and judgements are influenced by social factors, by other people. But there is something to be said in its favour.

1. It puts a high value on the personal experiences and judgements of individual patients. Only each patient can know what it is like to be in a particular predicament, experiencing particular care in a particular place at a particular time.

2. When samples of 'real' patients' experiences and views are elicited collectively and by suitable research methods, we can get a picture of to what extent 'ordinary', non-activist patients experience and value whatever aspect of care and of standards we are interested in: information, choice, respect, access, and so on (Chapter Ten). Activists in any social movement are different from non-activists. Non-activists are the majority, activists the minority. Activists can hold strange or dubious views that even their colleagues, let alone non-activists, would not accept. Perhaps some activists are too radical and extreme? Or too conservative and reactionary? Non-activists winnow radical views and gradually accept some of them (Chapter Eleven). So 'real' patients' collective views are essential for judging and thinking about healthcare.

3. In any case, dominant interest holders do not have to accept 'real' patients' views, whether idiosyncratic or in a majority. That is a privilege of dominance. Activists need not be discouraged by majority views contrary to their own. They know that social change takes time.

Looked at politically, however, the concept of the 'real' patient can help dominant interest holders to maintain their dominance.

1. Patients can speak only for themselves. If their views are sought as representative in any sense, they must be sought collectively, through sampling or in other ways (Chapters Five and Seven). In spite of this

obvious point, individual 'real' or 'ordinary' patients are sometimes appointed to advisory or policy-making groups, where they can have little effect (Williamson, 1998; Hogg and Williamson, 2001; Little et al, 2002; Learmonth et al, 2009).

2. Patients can only judge their conscious experiences. They will have missed any threats to their interests that took place while they were unconscious, from general anaesthesia, or in intensive care, for example. They will have missed any threats from policies or practices that were inadvertently or deliberately hidden from them (Chapter Two; Williamson, 2000a). Patient activists do not know about everything that goes on covertly; but they are likely to know more than 'real' patients do (Williamson, 2005).

3. 'Real' patients, like 'ordinary' lay people, will tend to accept dominant interest holders' views by default (Chapter Three). (This can be observed when 'real' patients take part in discussions in patient support groups, as well as following from Alford's theory.) The close link between knowledge and radicalness (Chapter Eight) is relevant here.

The confusion that surrounds 'real' patients allows professionals and corporate rationalisers to hold that individual 'real' patients' views are always more valid than those of activists. This belief can serve to repress patients' interests (above 1, 2, 3). Dominant interest holders find 'real' so useful that they apply it to other subordinate social groups.

◊◊ A black American academic said on BBC Radio 4 that she had been told "You're not a 'real' black – you speak like a white person" (31 May 2008). ◊◊

Some implications of radicalness and conservatism in doctors

The radical–conservative dimension or variable in doctors has significant implications and consequences for radical patient activism. Does this mean that radical patient activists can only make progress when their views and proposals meet with favour from radical doctors? No. The appeal of argument and evidence to the scientific side of medicine; good working relationships; the intelligence and goodwill of most doctors; individual doctors' conversion to more radical ways of thinking, their shifts along the conservative–radical continuum; the many personal, social and situational variables that affect doctors' responses to radical patient activism, and to the profession's own radical elements, come in.

Various groups of doctors and patients or patient activists now work together in various ways to formulate standards for treatment or research. Groups vary in what sorts of patients and health professionals take part and what their working arrangements are. But it is usually impossible to trace the radical–conservative dimension in the working groups from published accounts. In the next section, I give three examples of patient activists and doctors working together in patient liaison groups at the medical royal colleges. I was a member of each, so they are an insider's accounts, and pay attention to the radical–conservative dimension. Working together can be difficult; but it can achieve successes, as radical patient activists would define success. When it does, its influence can be powerful.

Patient liaison groups at the medical royal colleges

> *The first responsibility of the colleges is to raise standards of care for patients.*
>
> (Dr Michael Brindle, President of the Royal College of Radiologists, 1997, in Davies, 1997, p 3)

The first patient liaison group in a medical royal college was started at the Royal College of General Practitioners in 1983 by Dr John Lee, a GP, and Nancy Dennis, a patient activist (Dennis, 1988). The other medical royal colleges gradually followed, some hesitantly (Williamson, 2008c).

Patient liaison groups (PLGs) usually have roughly equal numbers of college medical members and 'lay' people, though sometimes lay people are a majority, 7 to 5 in the group at the Royal College of General Practitioners, 12 to 6 at the Royal College of Surgeons. A PLG is usually a subcommittees of its college council (governing body), which accepts or rejects its recommendations. The colleges pay expenses and sometimes honoraria for the lay members. Most colleges advertise for prospective lay members in the national press, shortlist and interview them. Most colleges appoint the medical members without a formal process (another double standard). The lay members' backgrounds are diverse. Some are radical or conservative patient activists, others may be corporate rationalisers or non-medical health professionals. The lay members' radical–conservative alignments, and the alignments of the medical members, are seldom known or deliberately chosen. In this section, I focus on the radical patient activist members among the lay members, though the other lay members affect discussions and decisions. Since the members are not in clinical relationships with each other and know nothing about each others' performances as patients or as clinicians, sensitive issues can be raised and discussed freely (Williamson, 1998).

Patient liaison group members comment on government documents, sit on other college committees, give talks at college conferences, and so on; but here I look only at their work on standards of care. Ideally, PLGs are partnerships between doctors and lay people in which they work together to define and promote high standards of care (Williamson, 1993; Wilkie, 1998). Like other partnerships, they can be fragile.

Patient activist members' and medical members' views may support, complement or conflict with each other. Many standards harbour potentially controversial issues, either self-evidently or when examined in detail. Then those issues must be explored in depth, with activist members gathering evidence and honing arguments, perhaps over many months. Those opposing the status quo of currently accepted standards have to work harder than those maintaining it: again we come back to Alford's observation that working for repressed interests requires much effort, for dominant interests, very little (Alford, 1975). But in order to achieve consensus over contested issues, dominant interest holders almost always have to concede more to repressed interest holders than vice versa (Chapter Two). The desirability, from the radical patient activists' perspective, of having at least one radical doctor among the medical members is obvious. Radical doctors are ready to argue against the conservatism of their medical colleagues. Radical doctors' arguments may also persuade conservative lay people to accept radical ideas more readily than radical patient activists' arguments can. (This is both an empirical observation and a theoretical point that follows from Chapter Three, the spread of radical ideas, and Chapter Five, the high status of clinicians' ideas.) Radical patient activists, however, can sometimes mobilise latent radical doctors' radicalness and so convert them into overt radicals, at least for some issues. A PLG depends on its medical members as much as on its lay members for its successful working (Williamson, 2008c).

Work on all three projects to be described in the next few pages required recurrent dialogue, negotiation and redrafting of texts over many months: conflict is inherent in the work. Indeed, unless some conflicts emerge, the patient members are possibly either inexperienced or are having difficulty voicing their views (Parroy et al, 2003). (Or all the medical and lay members are equally conservative or equally radical, see CHCs, Chapter Eight. But this is unlikely.) But even when radical ideas provoke insuperable opposition, the boundaries of discourse are enlarged, so that proposals unthinkable at first become accepted, sometimes without further debate, a few years later.

◊◊ The GP members of the Royal College of General Practitioners' PLG resisted the patient activists' suggestion that a range of self-help groups' pamphlets should be displayed in GPs' surgeries. The GPs said that they could only display pamphlets whose contents met with their entire approval. That was in 1992 (Williamson, 1993). Now patients sitting in their GPs' waiting rooms are surrounded by pamphlets and notices of helplines for a multitude of diseases. ◊◊

When a PLG sets out to formulate new standards of care for its college's specialty, it is in effect trying to change doctors' working arrangements or their clinical practice or both. PLGs can try to do this directly, through proposals intended to change professional behaviour, as in the first two examples described below. Or they can try to do it indirectly, through giving information to patients that implicitly sets out the standards they should expect, as in the third example.

Changing professional practice directly – the Royal College of General Practitioners (1997)

GPs have the right to remove patients, 'strike them off', from their personal lists (now practice lists) of patients, without warning or explanation, though patients are seldom told this until it happens to them.

◊◊ Of 320 leaflets of information for patients ('patient information') produced by general practices and current in 1995/96, only 3 mentioned the possibility of being struck off their GP's list (Royal College of General Practitioners, 1997a). ◊◊

None of the lay members had experienced being struck off. But they knew that patients were often extremely upset when it happened to them; that a new patient group, the Good Practice Campaign, had just been set up to oppose the practice; and that patients often called the Patients Association's helpline about it (Royal College of General Practitioners, 1997b). So the lay members raised the issue. Although the GP members were at first reluctant, they later took part enthusiastically, contributing instances of behaviour by GPs and by patients so bizarre that the lay members could not have imagined them.

All the PLG members agreed that there were some behaviours by patients that justified removal, like physical violence towards the GP, practice staff or other patients, or racist abuse. But some GPs struck patients off for reasons that should never justify removal: patients' decisions about clinical matters (requesting a home confinement, refusing cervical cytology screening, or immunisation for their children); or critical questions about the safety of practices (the sterilisation of instruments) or clinical techniques; or complaints. The PLG members agreed that a GP thinking about removing a patient from his or her list must: tell the patient that the GP sees a problem in the patient's behaviour; attempt to explain the GP's point of view; try to elicit the patient's perspective and interpretation; try to negotiate a new relationship with the patient, with concessions by both; and, if that fails, smooth the patient's path to a different GP in the same practice or in another practice (Royal College of General Practitioners, 1997b).

This proposal for change, this new standard, showed *respect* for patients. It supported *redress*: natural justice demands that people accused of bad behaviour must be told what is alleged against them. Attempts at reconciliation were relevant to *equity*, *access* and *choice*, especially as whole families were sometimes struck off because of the behaviour of one member. The college council accepted the PLG's policy paper and published it as guidance for college members in 1997 (Royal College of General Practitioners, 1997b).

Changing professional practice directly – the Royal College of Pathologists (2002)

Pathology laboratories send the results of routine tests, such as for cholesterol levels or viral loads for HIV in blood, and of diagnostic procedures, such as biopsies for suspected cancer, to the patient's GP or consultant. That clinician is then responsible for telling the patient. All the lay members of the Lay Advisory Committee (the patient liaison group) had experienced this system, some for routine biochemical results, others for diagnostic procedures. The patient activist members suggested that the results of routine pathology tests should be sent to patients direct from the laboratory. That would secure quicker test results for patients; fewer losses of results or failures to tell them to patients; removal of doubt about whether the patient or the clinician was responsible for ensuring that the patient got the results; and removal of ambiguity over whether 'no news is good news': this would improve *safety*. The full results, on paper or electronically, rather than an edited shorthand version ("your results are OK") would improve *information* and *safety*. Less time waiting for the results would reduce patients' anxiety and signify *respect*. Preventing patients from feeling demeaned and controlled, because other people knew something about them that they did not, would also signify *respect*.

The pathologist members of the Lay Advisory Committee agreed that routine test results should be sent direct to patients who wished to have them that way, with a copy to their clinician, if that were agreed by their clinician and the pathologist. (So patients would depend on that agreement; they were not entirely freed from their doctors' control over this information.) But the pathologists did not accept the patient activists' proposal that patients who wished to should also receive new diagnostic findings direct, although the arguments for this were at least as strong as those for test results. Many patients get extremely anxious, for example, when cancer is suspected, waiting several weeks, perhaps, for an appointment with their consultant. Some consultants refuse to release even negative results ('good news') over the telephone.

The Lay Advisory Group's paper was accepted by the college council in 2001 and its recommendations were included in college guidelines in 2002 (Crow, 2002). Like the pathologist members of the Lay Advisory Group, the college council rejected the idea that patients should receive diagnostic results direct. Council members said that it might undermine the relationship between patient and clinician, and that patients might not understand the significance of the results (Crow, 2002). (Attributing low abilities and unknown feelings to patients is oppressive, since it justifies treating them badly, Chapters One, Two and Five.)

This was an example of a step-wise sequence towards higher standards (Chapter Six). Patient activists secured the first step, routine test results, but not the second, new diagnostic results, though the issue, giving patient the *choice* of how and when they got *access* to their pathology results, was the same. Later research (unrelated to this project) showed that more patients wanted to get new diagnostic results from a health professional than wanted them direct. But both for routine tests and for diagnostic procedures, patients wanted to choose how to get the results (Pyper et al, 2004).

Information for patients and changing professional practice indirectly – the Royal College of Anaesthetists (2003)

At the Royal College of Anaesthetists, a working party of six anaesthetists and six radical patient activists produced a booklet for patients, *Anaesthesia explained*, as part of a wider project to raise the standards of information for patients about anaesthesia and anaesthetic practice (Royal College of Anaesthetists and Association of Anaesthetists of Great Britain and Ireland, 2002; Lack et al, 2003). *Anaesthesia explained* was intended to give patients the information they needed to play an informed part in their anaesthetic care. That entailed setting out explicitly the standards of care that patients should expect, so implicitly setting out the corresponding standards for anaesthetists' practice. The potential for conflict between patient activists and doctors was greater than in the other projects, partly because a much larger number of issues was covered, partly because information for patients is always liable to be contentious (Chapter Seven). All the patient activists had experienced having anaesthetics; but their knowledge had to extend far beyond the personal.

Patients about to undergo an anaesthetic need a lot of information in a short time, 'like reading a book on survival once the boat is sinking', said Dr Alastair Lack, the chair of the editorial board,(Lack, 2003, p 5). That meant the task of providing it was taxing and must be got right the first time. For *Anaesthesia explained*, almost every detail of content, level, explanation, tone and format was negotiated between the patient activist members and the medical members of the working party, at meetings or through series of e-mails (Lack, 2003).

◊◊ What the physiological state induced by general anaesthesia should be called was especially contentious, anaesthetists preferring 'sleep', patient activists, 'controlled unconsciousness' (Lack, 2003). Patient activists said that 'sleep' was misleading and patronising (Rollin, 2003). Anaesthetists said that they and their ('real') patients were happy with the word. (But their patients had probably only been offered the term 'sleep'.) The patient activists' preference prevailed in this publication, but not lastingly nor in the college. ◊◊

◊◊ Less contentious was the change activists wanted in the draft from 'the anaesthetist will only give you a blood transfusion if you need one' to '… if he or she thinks you need one'. The criteria for 'need' for transfusion changes with changing physiological knowledge and with patients' clinical states; and the revised wording could alert patients to ask their anaesthetist about this before the proposed operation. ◊◊

What is left out of information for patients can be as important as what is put in. Points excluded because the anaesthetists and the patient activists could not agree were usually those raised by the patient activists. Points that the anaesthetists wanted, but that the patient activists did not, were included, but worded with extra care. Compared with the number of points on which agreement was reached, the number of unresolved points and of omissions was small.

All the members of the working group were satisfied that high standards for *information, shared decision making* and *choice* were agreed. Points at which patients could make choices were flagged in the text. This extract on how clinical decisions are made and on shared decision making exemplifies the tone of the booklet:

◊◊ 'Having talked about the benefits, risks and your preferences, you can then decide together what would be best for you. Or you may prefer to ask your anaesthetist to decide for you. Nothing will happen to you until you understand and agree with what has been planned for you. You have the right to refuse if you do not want the treatment suggested. The choice of anaesthetic depends on:

- your operation
- your answers to the questions you have been asked [about your health]
- your physical condition
- your preferences and the reasons for them
- your anaesthetist's recommendations for you and the reasons for them
- the equipment, staff and other resources at your hospital.'

(Royal College of Anaesthetists and Association of Anaesthetists of Great Britain and Ireland, 2003, p 13) ◊◊

This, adapted for other treatments and situations, is a model for all clinical decision making in which patients can take part. It could reassure those who wished to make an autonomous choice of dependency that the decisions made for them had been thought through thoroughly. It could enable those who wished to explore or question their doctor's advice to do so in a logical way that would not imply that the patient distrusted the doctor.

Points arising from the three projects

The roughly equal numbers of doctors and patient activists in the groups working on these projects made them unusual; many groups that advise on or set standards are multidisciplinary, with radical (or any) patient activists in a minority. The compositions of these three groups made tensions over political, cultural and emotional issues clear.

Political

Political tensions arose from members' assumptions about the purposes of their work. Members could see their work predominantly (a) as educating patients or (b) as empowering them (Dixon-Woods, 2001). ('Empowerment' means making the balance of power between professional and patient more equal, redressing the imbalance (Gilbert, 1995).) They could see their work predominantly (a) as giving information to patients or (b) as changing professional practice. In addition, members could see lay people's views on clinical or technical matters (a) as illegitimate invasions of professional territory or (b) as legitimate. And they could see clinicians' views on non-clinical and psychosocial issues (a) as valid or (b) as sometimes questionable.

The more radical the patient activist and the doctor members were, the more likely they were to take the (b) positions in these sets of pairs. These dichotomies are over-simplified but they indicate why stressful disagreements could arise. These disagreements were especially intense because the assumptions or convictions that lay under them were seldom put into explicit words.

Cultural

Any social group's culture, its accustomed ways of thinking and feeling about itself and about social groups outside itself, unites and influences the group's members. Doctors' medical culture is strong and pervades all that doctors do (Irvine, 2003; Jorm and Kam, 2004). In these three projects, the medical members seldom denied the validity of what the patient activist members said, once they adduced their evidence and arguments. Conflicts over what to include or exclude usually sprang from the medical members' caution about what their medical peers outside the group would think. Would different policies, practices or standards disrupt established working arrangements and relationships? Or clinical relationships between clinician and patient? Were some proposed standards 'too high' for current practice, even though the medical members agreed with them personally? Would including them make other doctors dismiss the patient information booklets as unfeasible or absurd? Would including them be 'telling other doctors what to do', that is, failing to respect their clinical autonomy? This last reason for excluding a proposed new policy or new standard fits with doctors' defence of each other's clinical autonomy, and disinclination to influence other doctors' clinical practice (Armstrong and Ogden, 2006).

These arguments were difficult for patient activists to counter. If dominant interest holders say "we can't do it", they take advantage of their strong position, if their work is valued or needed by society, or if they can persuade society that it is (Chapter Two).

Emotional

Discussing standards of care is always demanding and stressful, because standards of care evoke strong feelings in both doctors and patients.

Doctors take pride in their profession and want to believe that what they do, the standards that they work to, are good and right. Doctors' sense of self-esteem may be threatened if the standards to which they personally work are criticised, even if no one else in the group knows what those standards are. "As humans, we have to believe we are right and have to continue with it, even if it is shown to be wrong," said Dr C. Patient activists also believe that they are right in pressing for changes to standards. But they know that they may need medical care sometime. So they may feel that their survival could be threatened by low standards, sometimes their physical survival, sometimes their survival as moral agents (Chapter Four). Threats to self-esteem or to survival, not necessarily consciously felt, can prompt primitive levels of thinking and functioning (Halton, 1994). Bad behaviour in patient liaison groups both by lay people and by doctors – threats to resign; frequent absences from meetings; accounts of one's own clinical practice as a doctor or of one's own clinical experience as a patient that are intended to silence discussion rather than to add to it – are not unknown.

Connected to self-esteem, and to concern about their livelihoods, doctors' fear of patients' complaints can be intense (Allsop and Mulcahy, 1999). That fear can carry over into PLGs at national level (Dr A, personal communication, 2004). Such fear seems irrational to the lay members because working relationships are different from clinical relationships. But patient activists can have reciprocal fears: they can fear the disgrace of the college abolishing its patient liaison group. In reality, two PLGs have been threatened with abolition. Both survived.

Nevertheless, doctors and patient activists can easily imagine each other as more persecutory than they actually are.

On the other hand, doctors and patient activists can feel great cordiality towards each other, confident of mutual understanding and support. Nevertheless, patient activists and doctors have to learn to manage their feelings of ambivalence towards each other in working relationships, just as they have to in clinical ones (Williamson, 2001).

Good working relationships are fundamental to this work. They make frank discussion possible. In particular, when good working relationships and trust are established, medical members sometimes tell activists about practices or professional assumptions that the activists could not have discovered for themselves.

◊◊ It was a haematologist who told me about some hospitals withholding the national leaflets on blood transfusion (Chapter Six), taking me aside after a meeting to express his concern. ◊◊

Sometimes doctors feel that an issue is too sensitive or too radical to raise openly with their peers. Then they hope that activists will find a way of calling attention to it. ("Thank goodness you said that!" is a common private response to something an activist has said.) Or sometimes an issue is so controversial within the specialty that the medical members welcome patient activists' views. Reciprocally, activists can alert doctors to new issues emerging from patients' experiences. Or they can give doctors new insights.

◊◊ "You make me think" or "I have learned such a lot from all of you" are commonly said to patient activists by doctors who have worked with them. ◊◊

Political, cultural and emotional tensions make discussions about standards of care strategically and emotionally exacting. Activists can feel that they are walking on a tightrope that they will fall off if they are too radical and demanding or too conservative and undemanding. Even when activists are demanding, they seldom secure as many steps as they would like in the sequences towards the ever-higher standards that they envisage (Chapter Six). Doctors, contrariwise, can feel they have agreed to things that they should not have (medical member of a PLG, personal communication, 2004).

Purposes and interests

In spite of frustrations and doubts, all the members of a PLG can feel that dialogue and negotiation can achieve progress towards higher standards. Sometimes doctors accept patient activists' appeals to the ethical or clinical values of the medical profession.

> ◊ ◊ GPs accepted that the patients should have access to their medical records as a support for their autonomy, not to encourage their compliance with treatment (Williamson, 1993). ◊ ◊

More often, a form of words can be agreed because it meets both doctors' and patient activists' interests and purposes, although they are different. Part of activists' task is to argue that professionals' and patients' interests, once they have been identified and explained in discussion, can sometimes be made compatible with each other (Williamson, 1992). Interests are many faceted, and activists' arguments can sometimes alter the relative values doctors put on the facets.

> ◊ ◊ Some anaesthetists thought that patients should not be told about autologous blood transfusion (Chapter Six) if it were not provided in their hospital, because that could reduce patients' confidence in the hospital and in them. The arguments in the example in Chapter Six (pp 104-5) changed their minds. ◊ ◊

But doctors' and patient activists' purposes can remain different.

> ◊ ◊ Anaesthetists and patient activists agreed that patients should be told in detail what to expect during anaesthetic procedures. This can be seen as education: patients will understand and cooperate with what will happen (Smith, 2003). Or it can be seen as empowerment: patients will be able to question the procedure, ask for it to be modified, and refuse or accept it from an informed position (Smith, 2003). ◊ ◊

Preserving differences in purpose and perspective ensures that agreement is based neither on the domination of activists by their medical colleagues nor on their cooptation. Resistance to domination is necessary for social change (Touraine, 1995). Achieving harmony over an issue can alter the balance of power in patients' favour without evoking intractable resistance from doctors. Cumulatively, this can add up to significant changes. Compromise, often recommended for negotiations in general, should probably be the last resort when the parties are markedly different in power (Parroy et al, 2003).

Differences in purpose and perspective are worth keeping, even emphasising. Radical activists have no wish to undermine doctors' professionalism, any more than they wish to turn into quasi-doctors themselves. They wish to support what is valuable about the profession and its specialties, while freeing patients from coercion and institutionalised disadvantage (Chapter One).

Conclusion

Radical and conservative alignments and positions in doctors are important, as they are in patient activists. Doctors and activists working together can articulate new standards successfully. But the emotional, cultural and political implications of alliances and antagonisms have been little thought about. Without thorough analyses, rigorous and sympathetic to the positions and feelings of all parties, it will remain hard for the royal colleges and other institutions or groups to set and to secure the implementation of the high standards that should characterise healthcare.

TEN

Achievements and failures

Two steps forward and one step backwards – or is it one step forward and two steps backwards?

(Ann Seymour, radical patient activist, 2006, personal communication)

Introduction

Tracing and assessing radical patient activism's successes and failures in opposing specific widely accepted policies, practices and standards and in securing higher ones is difficult. Its successes become absorbed into taken-for-granted practice. Proposed new standards are accepted or rejected at different rates in different places (Williamson, 1987), and some of radical patient activism's failures eventually become successes. This chapter looks at the origins of some standards and at the influence of patient activism's principles on other people concerned with healthcare: patients, health professionals, corporate rationalisers and reformers unconnected with the patient movement. It then looks at radical activists' effects on standards of care. Influences and effects are closely connected, since patient activists can only bring about change through corporate rationalisers and health professionals. In addition, corporate rationalisers and professionals are affected by ideas and circumstances that are independent of patient activism and of patients' views and wishes.

Tracing the origins of new standards

Standards are the values given to practices; they are ideas. Disentangling any single individual's or social group's ideas from the others' and from the swarm of ideas and sensibilities around at the time, the *zeitgeist*, is often impossible. Different people may have had the same idea at about the same time (Chapter Three; Pierson, 2004). Then, who first accepted a new practice or standard and caused it to be introduced into professional or institutional practice can be hard to pinpoint. Patient groups and individual activists are at a disadvantage here because their ideas and proposed standards can easily be attributed to more powerful or more conspicuous people.

1. Patient groups' accounts of what they think and do are often published in the 'grey' literature, that is, in publications like patient groups' journals which do not qualify for inclusion in MEDLINE or other databases. So other patient groups, health professionals, researchers, social scientists and commentators can find it difficult to discover work by patient groups and patient activists. The patient movement lacks a journal comparable with reputable healthcare professional journals, in which proposed new standards can be flagged up and debated (Chapter Two).

2. Obviously, patient activists cannot directly introduce new ways of doing things into professionals' practice. Activists have no test beds to try out new varieties of seedlings. They cannot introduce a new practice or standard, then write it up to show that it is feasible and that it benefits patients. Their success in introducing a new standard usually has to come through professionals (Chapter Nine). Patient activists can press ideas and proposed standards on national and local professional or corporate rationalist organisations. But they, too, then have to work through individual health professionals as dominant interest holders, who are in a position to disregard corporate rationalisers' and patient activists' views and wishes (Chapter Two).

3. Dominant interest holders readily take other groups' ideas and knowledge without acknowledging where they got them from. They can 'delete the original authorship of the lay public from the acknowledged history' of a disease or condition (Arksey, 1994, p 464).

    ◊◊ The effect of RAGE in improving standards of radiotherapy 'got no recognition from anyone, professional, political or legal' (Chapter Five). ◊◊

4. Alternatively, dominant interest holders can disregard subordinate groups' ideas and knowledge. Or see them as trivial or as subversive.

    ◊◊ Men literary critics have habitually omitted women's novels, poems and literary criticism from anthologies and university courses (Felski, 2003). Feminist criticism has developed as a counter-sensibility, which has then often met with masculine hostility (Felski, 2003). Similarly, professionals and corporate rationalisers have tended to disregard the 'patient perspective' or counter-sensibility. Or they have seen articulate patients or patient activists as selfish or as doctor bashers (Chapters Seven and Nine). ◊◊

3 and 4 reflect dominant interest holders' power to decide what counts and what does not count. To health professionals, patient groups and individual patients can seem invisible and voiceless. (But having their voices ignored can prompt repressed interest holders to become radical, Chapter Four.)

5. When professionals come to understand the reasons for the standards for which radical patient activists have pressed, they may feel that their own practice could have harmed their patients. It is hard to live with remorse. Professionals may deny their guilt by believing that their practice was better than it was or that they changed it earlier than they did.

> ◊◊ Some paediatricians have recently claimed that they introduced unrestricted parental visiting into their wards some years before NAWCH surveys showed that they did (Peg Belson, personal communication, 2008). ◊◊

Patient activists want to see new standards adopted quickly. One of their reasons, though one tinged with self-interest, is a wish to spare professionals the pain of guilt for not having acted earlier.

6. We all tend to attribute good ideas and successful achievements more generously to ourselves than to other people who were, or who might have been, also involved. (In sociology, this generalisation is called 'attribution theory'.)

Overlooking the contributions of patient activism to ideas and standards of care has various consequences. For one thing, health professionals may have little sense of the continuities and of the directions of changes to standards of care (Chapter Six). When patient activists press for a new higher standard, professionals can feel as if an arbitrary attack or an unwarranted demand is being made upon their values and their professionalism, '... meddling with how doctors behave and think', to quote an anaesthetist (Hooper, 2008, p 2472). Resentment probably increases some doctors' resistance to the standards that patient activists propose.

For another thing, neglecting to refer to relevant research or other work published by patient groups makes it look as if all improvements in healthcare are entirely due to professionals. This falsifies history. It can also exclude relevant ideas and experiences from professionals' and corporate rationalisers' thoughts and discussions. Above all, it is repressive.

> ◊◊ A colloquium of 'leading improvement practitioners, healthcare managers, clinicians and policy makers in the UK', meeting to discuss ways of improving healthcare, suggested that improvements might be brought about by (a non-existent) social movement among healthcare staff (Bate et al, 2004, p 62). 'Social movements theory' was discussed but no mention was made of the patient movement. ◊◊

In spite of problems with attribution, we can sometimes partly trace the spread and acceptance of patient radicalism's ideas.

The spread of radical patient activism's principles

The principles that radical patient activism espouses are now widely accepted. Principles, like other ideas, spread through various social communications and relationships that may give them different meanings. But some commonality of meaning remains (Chapters Six and Seven).

The patient movement as a whole

Patient support groups, as well as radical activist groups, have long wanted better information for patients (Wilson, 2005). Most patient groups now emphasise the importance of choice, access and equity as well as of information (Baggott et al, 2005). Although most patient groups are conservative at any given time, most probably gradually adopt some radical ideas (Chapter Three). Whether they take them from radical patient groups or from the *zeitgeist* or from professionals who have begun to accept them probably varies. Strongly conservative patient groups probably tend to accept once-radical ideas only after professionals have accepted them (Chapter Three).

◊ ◊ There was evidence from my CHC research that CHC members who were not members of radical patient groups used common-sense knowledge to judge standards of care (Chapter Eight). Common-sense or lay knowledge is sometimes yesterday's professional knowledge (Chapter Five). ◊◊

The International Alliance of Patients' Organizations believes that patient care must be based on five principles: respect; choice for patients and empowerment for patient organisations; patients' and patients' organisations' involvement in health policy; access and support; and information (www.patientsorganizations.org). Other patient organisations cite various mixes of the same or similar principles.

Patients

How far do 'ordinary' or 'real' patients share the ideas and principles of the patient activists who profess to speak for their interests? Non-activist patients have benefited from the activities of activists, just as 'ordinary' women have benefited from the activities of feminists, 'ordinary' black people from those of black activists. But have patient activism's principles spread to non-activists? Or have activists abstracted principles from what patients say about their experiences? Probably both (Chapter Six). Evidence that patients' unarticulated or tacit principles are similar to activists' articulated ones comes from surveys of patients' views and through patient involvement.

Surveys

Surveys of large samples of patients can give a picture of how they judge the extent to which information, choice, shared decision making and so on were offered to them. Surveys repeated over time can measure shifts in patients' judgements of care, though how far they reflect changes in the standards of care patients experience, and how far changes in patients' responses to them, is often uncertain. Questions in surveys are sometimes inexact or superficial (Chapter Five). Even so, surveys can give insights into patients' judgements, not so much about the principles themselves as about practices and standards that can be related to those principles.

◊ ◊ National surveys in England, conducted by Picker Institute Europe on samples of tens of thousands of patients and repeated every year, found that in 2006:

- 92% of general practice patients and 78% of hospital in-patients patients said they were always treated respectfully;
- 79% of patients said they were 'given the right amount' of information before treatment, 84% before anaesthesia;
- 79% of general practice patients said they had been given enough information about the purpose of any medicine prescribed for the first time for them, 76% of hospital patients;
- 58% of general practice patients and 37% of hospital patients said they were told enough or 'completely' about their medicines' side effects;
- 55% of general practice patients had taken part in deciding about what medicine they should take;
- 48% of hospital patients said they had not been involved in decisions about their care as much as they wanted to be;
- 42% of patients said they were given information about how to look after themselves at home;
- 37% of hospital in-patients had received copies of the correspondence about them between their GP and their specialist, 25% of out-patients;
- 32% of general practice patients said they had not been involved in decisions about their care as much as they wanted to be (Richards and Coulter, 2007). ◊◊

Data like these are difficult to interpret. But they indicate that large numbers of patients are not satisfied with the amount of *information* and *shared decision making* offered them.

Patient involvement

The terms 'patient involvement' or 'patient participation' are used both for individual patients engaging with health professionals, for example, in shared decision making, and for patients whose views professionals and corporate rationalisers seek through relationships that are outside the clinical relationship. The second meaning is the one used here.

Involvement is like patient activism in that both entail discussion between dominant and repressed interest holders. They differ in that, in involvement, dominant interest holders take the initiative and invite patients to take part; in activism, patient activists take the initiative and try to gain dominant interest holders' attention. In involvement, dominant interest holders select the patients to be involved; set the agenda; sometimes provide information and opinion; and control the boundaries round the topics or issues being discussed. In activism, activists choose which dominant interest holders to approach; ask or apply to take part in discussions; set the agenda or raise issues that are not on the dominant interest holders' agenda; bring with them their own new knowledge; and try to push at the boundaries of what dominant interest holders will accept.

Involvement takes many forms and addresses many topics, from standards of care and planning future services to prioritising some forms of care over others. From the mass of data that involvement generates, patients' support for activism's principles and desire for higher standards of care can sometimes be discerned.

> ◊◊ Exploring patients' experiences of treatment and care for cancers of the head and neck showed staff that patients felt unsafe on a post-surgical ward because staff and visitors did not always wash their hands (Bate and Robert, 2007). (Here the principle was *safety*.) ◊◊

Involvement and patient activism, whether conservative or radical activism, should probably be seen as complementary to each other, with some overlaps in practice. Inviting activists to take part in deciding what issues to ask patients about, for example, can be useful in drawing dominant interest holders' attention to aspects of care that they might have not have considered (Thornton et al, 2003). Involvement can be especially important when it includes patients who have no patient groups to speak for their perceptions, values and interests. But however extensively and sensitively involvement is undertaken, it and activism are alike in one way: dominant interest holders have the power to disregard what either involved patients or patient activists say.

Health professionals

The principles of radical patient activism are supported by many doctors (Smith, 2003). But doctors differ from each other in what standards they choose to work to. Dr Smith's list of practices in order of anaesthetists' probable resistance to them (Chapter Six, p 101) was an example. Some anaesthetists were willing to offer certain *choices* to patients, others were not. Not offering choice for a practice for which choice is feasible is a standard whose value is 'no choice'. But professionals do not always see negative values for standards as consciously chosen standards rather than as just a routine part of the way things are done. They may need a radical fellow professional or a radical patient activist to point that out to them, to 'raise their consciousness', in the language of emancipation movements.

On the other hand, sometimes professionals subscribe to a principle, like some midwives to informed *choice*, so idealistically that they seem scarcely to notice that their own practice denies it (Hindley and Thomson, 2005). Or they subscribe to a principle but are uncertain how far to express it in the values they attach to practices. How much to tell patients about a specific practice or course of action is a problem for professionals, even when they have willingly accepted *information* as a principle. The range between 'as little as possible' and 'everything' is large (Chapter Seven). 'As little as possible' is the least amount necessary for patients to consent to (or refuse) some proposed course of action. It is the weakest expression of the principle. 'Everything' is the principle's strongest expression. Offering no information at all denies the principle.

Again, patient activists can sometimes point out discrepancies between principles and the actual standards in place, so helping professionals to meet their own aspirations to practise their professions well. Discrepancies are not always a source of conflict between professionals and activists, for some professionals welcome activists' ability to see things in healthcare that they, the professionals, do not (Chapter Nine).

Corporate rationalisers

The Department of Health, acting for the government, also uses the words *information, choice, safety, shared decision making*, and *patient autonomy*. But exactly what they mean is often doubtful because publications from the Department tend to be high in rhetoric and low in analytic precision or explanation. Ambiguities, inconsistencies and lack of definitions characterise corporate rationalisers' pronouncements (Alford, 1975). These bureaucratic devices make it easy for corporate rationalisers to look good, but to ditch their policies if they are intractably opposed by doctors or if they prove too costly.

The NHS Plan of 2000 promised more *information*, wider *choices*, more *involvement in decision making* about treatment and a better system of *redress* (Department of Health, 2000). But the Department of Health may fail to secure standards that it knows patients would like, as in Example 1. Or it may rescind established standards that patients value and expect, as in Example 2.

◊◊ *Example 1.* The 2001 Health and Social Care Act proposed that patients would get copies of the letters about them between their GP and their hospital consultant (Lister, 2004). In 2002, the Department of Health said that this would be implemented by 2004 (Lister, 2004). But the medical profession opposed the practice and succeeded in stopping its implementation (Lister, 2004). Some consultants send copies to patients, others do not, even in the same hospital (personal observation, 2009). ◊ ◊

◊ ◊ *Example 2*. The Department of Health has allowed primary care trusts to abolish the long-standing 'right' of patients, with their GP, to choose the named hospital consultant to whom they wish to be referred (Elliot-Smith, 2009). Corporate rationalisers' interests in using doctors' time efficiently have overridden rhetoric about choice and made healthcare more impersonal. ◊ ◊

The Department's mixed positions towards patients' interests, sometimes promoting them, sometimes undermining them, are replicated at local trust level by executive managers. What actions managers take depends on their political and pragmatic priorities. Not annoying doctors or upsetting staff, when there are more important battles to win than securing the standards of care that patient activists want, is managers' overriding priority (chief executive of an NHS trust, personal communication, 1996).

◊ ◊ Meeting managerial targets was thought to be a factor that contributed to poor treatment and care at Stafford Hospital, where the Healthcare Commission investigated the high death rates of patients admitted as emergencies from 2005 to 2008 (Healthcare Commission, 2009). To meet a target that patients should not stay in the Accident and Emergency Department for more than 4 hours, some patients were moved to a 'clinical decision unit', where they were sometimes left without monitoring or care (Healthcare Commission, 2009; Chapter Two). ◊ ◊

Other organisations

Various other organisations, concerned with healthcare but unconnected with the patient movement, have adopted some of the same principles, though their ideologies differ from those of radical patient activism. Humane care and patient-centred care, for example, share some principles with radical patient activism. But their theoretical approaches are different. Humane care (Chochinov, 2007; Pellegrino and Thomasma, 1981) is doctor centred and doctor aligned. Patient-centred care (Gerteis et al, 1993; Picker Institute, 2007) is patient centred and corporate rationaliser aligned. Neither includes patient autonomy among the values and principles it espouses. Another difference is that they see good care as something given to patients by staff. Radical patient activists see many aspects of good care like that, as well. But they also see some aspects of good care as care in which staff have not denied patients something that belongs to them, their autonomy. The difference in day-to-day practice may often be slight; but the difference in philosophy is great.

The spread of radical standards

Dominant interest holders can harm repressed interest holders innocently or inadvertently, without realising the effects of their actions upon them (Chapter Two). Conversely, doctors can introduce practices and standards into their work that benefit patients by supporting their autonomy, although the doctors' purposes are to secure some other benefit.

> ◊◊ In 1925, Sir James Spence took mothers to live-in in the Babies' Hospital at Newcastle, so that they could continue to breast-feed (Hales-Tooke, 1973). ◊◊

> ◊◊ In 1927, Dr and Mrs Pickerill took mothers to live-in in a plastic surgery unit in Wellington, New Zealand, to reduce cross-infection (Hales-Tooke, 1973). ◊◊

These practices predated NAWCH by almost 30 years. But they set precedents for mothers to live-in with their babies and young children. They showed that it was feasible and could benefit patients.

A more recent example comes from pathology.

> ◊◊ In 2005, pathologists in one hospital invited patients who had had hysterectomies for benign conditions to come to the pathology department to look at their diseased uteri, removed during surgery (Hock et al, 2005). The pathologists intended this to help patients understand why they had been advised to have a hysterectomy and to show them that retaining excised tissue was valuable for research (Hock et al, 2005). ◊◊

Patient activists welcome this new practice because it respects some patients' wish to see their excised body parts; gives them extra information about their clinical state; and can add to their understanding of their situation.

Practices and standards that meet the wishes and purposes both of clinicians and of patient activists can be accommodated in practices and standards of healthcare without conflict. Just as activists' and professionals' different perspectives and purposes can sometimes be met within a single form of words, when they write patient information together, a harmony of interests has been attained (Chapter Nine). These harmonies can be small but significant steps in the direction of shared power and equality.

Figure 10.1 shows the typical career of a new standard, from its origin to its acceptance or rejection by dominant interest holders. Patient activists come to feel uneasy about a current practice or standard, perhaps after patients have told them about it, perhaps from their own experience, observation or reading (Chapter Five). They put into words a better standard, as they define better, and put the new one forward to dominant interest holders. Ideas from any source, including from health professionals, can be drawn in at any stage in the process.

Figure 10.1: Stages from total repression to emancipation

1. Patients and patient activists accept dominant definitions
of patients' interests
↓
2. Patients and patient activists identify conflict of interests –
may form a patient group
↓
3. Patient group works on issue
↓
4. Patient activists begin to get issue into the public arena,
including to other patients
↓
5. Patients' and patient activists' views not heard
↓
6. Views heard but not accepted
↓
7. Views heard and considered
↓
8. Patients' and patients' views prevail or fail to prevail then,
but may succeed later

Each step may be fraught with frustration and anguish, or may prove unexpectedly easy.

This model can probably fit any emancipation movement, provided it allows for ideas from various radical sources to be included at every stage. The model moves from the complete repression of repressed interest holders' interests; through their partial repression; to their release from repression through the articulation of new ways of doing things; to argument and pressure to get dominant interest holders to accept them. The middle stages of awareness and struggle are likely to be experienced by repressed interest holders as oppression. But during the first stage, when repressed interest holders' interests are so completely repressed that they are unaware that they even have an interest in the practice or standard, all seems calm and 'natural' (Chapter Two). These first stages constitute the 'false consciousnesses' or 'latent interests' noted in Chapter Two.

◊◊ There were fewer women's than men's colleges in Oxford in the early and mid 20th century, so young women had a worse chance of gaining a place at that university than did young men. Women's disadvantage seemed 'natural'; women were probably less academic than men. Then the men's colleges started to admit women; and now colleges, including the former women's colleges, admit both women and men. ◊◊

The progress of patient activism's emancipatory ideas can be examined in two ways: by their effects on health professionals and by their effects on standards of care.

Assessing progress: radical patient activists' influence on health professionals

What causes doctors to resist changing their behaviour or to accept it has been much studied (Lomas, 1993; Greco and Eisenberg, 1993). A change usually requires a combination of motivating factors that may include the influence of local colleagues, new regulations from corporate rationalisers, public policy, professional bodies, financial incentives, insurance companies, patient groups and individual patients, and wider external factors like technological and economic circumstances (Lomas, 1993). Local colleagues are especially important (Lomas, 1993). Patient pressure groups can be influential because they are knowledgeable, concerned and committed; but they often lack resources and may lack credibility in doctors' eyes (Lomas, 1993; Chapter Five).

◊◊ A formerly conservative, now radical, paediatric anaesthetist had long held out against pressure to allow parents into the anaesthetic room until their child became unconscious. He told me that he had made the change from preventing parents from coming into the anaesthetic room to allowing them there for four reasons:

1. Technical advances meant that heavy pre-medication was no longer given in the ward, where the parents were beside their child until the child was asleep, but was given more lightly, or not at all, in the anaesthetic room, where the child was conscious and, unless a parent were there, crying.
2. He went to a talk about the issue by a NAWCH member ("NAWCH was revolutionary at the time," he said).
3. An educational psychologist on the hospital staff kept asking him, when they met in the corridors, when he was going to change the policy.
4. Anaesthetists in other London hospitals were doing it.

"We were dragged into it," he said. (Eminent paediatric anaesthetist, personal communication, 2008) ◊◊

Health professionals who consult or collaborate with radical patient groups 'gradually become more radical, though that may require changes in well-established policies and practices' (Durward and Evans, 1990, p 270). Put the other way round, professionals who, for whatever reasons, accept policies, practices or standards advocated by radical patient groups or activists, probably become more radical than before towards future controversial standards. They can change from taking predominantly conservative positions to taking more radical ones (Chapter Nine). Whether they change because they come to understand the activists' reasons for the new policies, practices and standards or because they come to like and respect the patient activists with whom they work is unclear; probably both (Chapter Nine).

There are, it goes without saying, many examples of professionals, like the paediatrician and ward sisters in York in the 1960s (Chapter Five), who remain unmoved by radical patient activists' best efforts. Or professionals go some, but only some, way towards meeting activists' desired standards (Chapter Nine).

Assessing progress: activists' effects on standards of care

Radical patient activists reflecting on changes to standards of patient care over the last 40 or 50 years, since the mid-1960s, would probably judge that in many ways they have improved. Information for patients, for example, is fuller and deals with clinical matters, not just visiting times and 'bring your own toothbrush'.

Some standards have improved so much that few people remember that once they were different. Parents with their children in paediatric wards might be surprised to hear that it took more than 30 years of unremitting effort to achieve freedom from coercively restrictive visiting for every parent and child in the UK. But some standards remain low, after many years of activists' efforts. Others have worsened. At the same time, new policies that threaten patients' interests are incorporated into practice, often without patients or patient activists knowing anything about them until they are in place.

◊◊ In general practice, getting to the surgery and getting to see a particular GP has become more difficult than it was 60 years ago (Wilkie, 2008). This reduced *access* prevents patient and doctor from building up a relationship in which each knows the strengths, weaknesses and idiosyncrasies of the other and on which they can base a therapeutic partnership. Impairing patients' ability to manage their consultations with their GP undermines their autonomy and the kind of shared decision making described in Chapter Seven. ◊◊

Occasionally, too, standards are deliberately lowered.

◊◊ Cutting back visiting times in adult wards in York Hospital in the early 2000s is an example (Chapter Seven, p 129). ◊◊

Progress, stasis and regression can probably be traced in every specialty. Maternity care is a good example because practices and standards in it have probably been more thoroughly and repeatedly scrutinised by radical patient activists and by radical health professionals than in any other specialty (with the possible exception of psychiatric care).

Maternity care

Patient activists in maternity care have played a crucial part in many western countries (Wagner, 1994). They have been catalysts for change, bringing together different groups of people and organising effective public campaigns. 'They are the unsung heroes of the change process' (Wagner, 1994, p 326). Yet AIMS judges that some policies, practices and standards in maternity care in the UK are worse than before (Beech, 2005).

Maternity care, though professing to meet the needs and wishes of each woman ('individualised' or 'patient-centred' care), readily slips into routines. Routines suit staff. They are desirable also for some aspects of complex care because they can provide a basic level of safety. But routine practices can become so taken for granted by staff that they forget to ask for each patient's consent to them. So routines become compulsory unless individual patients refuse them, evade them or successfully ask for something else. Routine practices that have no benefits under the circumstances in which they are used, or whose benefits are outweighed by their risks of harm, are ethically doubtful. That they are compulsory unless successfully opposed makes them coercive, a denial of patient autonomy. If patients cannot oppose them because they are unaware of them (because they are not disclosed to them or because they are treated as part of 'normal' care), they are strongly coercive (Chapter Two). (A compulsory practice that has high benefits and low or no risks of harm is still coercive; but, provided patients are aware of and accept the reasons for it, is not necessarily ethically wrong. The law of the land is coercive in this sense, but citizens know what it is and usually comply with it; most of us obey traffic lights, even if there is no other traffic.)

AIMS notes that some of the harsh and inhumane practices it opposed in the 1960s, 1970s and 1980s have gone (Chapter Four). Gone too are some clinical practices that AIMS opposed, including routine showers, enemas and pubic shaves at the beginning of labour; induction at 38 weeks of pregnancy; and routine episiotomies (Wright, 2003/4; Beech, 2004/5). None of these practices was justified by evidence; some caused harm to women and babies; and all caused distress to many women (Enkin et al, 1989).

The new knowledge that AIMS has created; AIMS' ability to discern flaws in scientific and social research; its criticisms of professionals' practices and standards; its warnings against the indiscriminate or routine use of non-clinical and clinical interventions; its good relationships with radical obstetricians, GPs, midwives and researchers;

its responses to Department of Health documents; its membership of the Royal College of Obstetricians and Gynaecologists' Consumer Group (a patient liaison group); its members' writings in professional journals and the popular media; its members' work on local health service governance bodies and other committees, all probably played a part in bringing about changes. Effort does not guarantee success; but without effort, there can be no success.

AIMS has so far been unsuccessful in opposing the routine use of obstetric interventions, like caesarean sections for breech births, that can sometimes be avoided by skilled care (Enkin et al, 1990). The routine use of technological interventions in low-risk women continues to worry AIMS. There is no evidence of their benefit and some evidence of their harm (Beech, 2005).

In addition, new technologies bring new ethical hazards or revive old ones. In the 1960s and 1970s, there were relatively few variations in patterns of midwifery and obstetric care. Then new technologies (machines, anaesthetic and other drugs) increased the number of patterns of care that could be provided by health professionals and chosen by women. New technological practices can benefit care, making it safer for women and foetuses at risk, and enabling women to choose the kind of care that best meets their views of their responsibilities for their baby, themselves and their families. But the large number of possible patterns of care has led some midwives to withhold information about those that they or the local obstetricians cannot or do not choose to provide. Some midwives have used new technologies and information about them to control women coercively, rather than to support their autonomy.

◊◊ Midwives in some maternity units did not offer women copies of the Midwives Information and Resource Service, MIDIRS, leaflets that described evidence-based patterns of care and the pros and cons of each, based on research, to help women make their own choices (Stapleton et al, 2002). MIDIRS leaflets, first issued in 1996 and since updated, cover issues like support in labour; monitoring the baby in labour; ultrasound in early pregnancy; alcohol; positions in labour and delivery; place of birth (home or hospital); management of breech presentation; and screening for congenital abnormality (MIDIRS and the NHS Centre for Reviews and Dissemination, 1996). ◊◊

Similarly, midwives sometimes deliberately bias the information they offer women, guiding their choices towards the midwives' or the obstetricians' personal preferences or the unit's policies.

◊◊ In one study, midwives steered women towards accepting continuous electronic monitoring by machine instead of intermittent monitoring by instruments held in the midwife's hands (Hindley and Thomson, 2005). Electronic monitoring turns the delivery room into an intensive care unit and increases the risk of false alarms about the foetus's heart rate and so can lead to 'unnecessary' caesarean sections (Enkin et al, 1990). ◊◊

Even for basic choices, distorted or misleading information has been given to women.

◊◊ "'You can choose to have your baby at home – providing a midwife is available" – what women are not told is that a midwife is always available because the Trust has a [legal] obligation to provide one.' (Beech, 2005, p 3) ◊◊

Thus, maternity care still shows that obstetricians and midwives, as dominant interest holders, can act coercively towards repressed interest holders, sometimes at the expense of their physical welfare, as well as of their autonomy. This coercion is not simply due to obstetricians favouring a medical model of childbirth while many women favour a social model of childbirth. Medical models can include information, choice and so on, just as much as social models; and social models can be coercive.

Accidental poor care and low standards

Accidentally poor care has to be distinguished from accepted low standards of treatment and care, as patient activists would define low. Making that distinction can be difficult without detailed knowledge of what current professional standards should be. Professionals reviewing each others' practices and standards are an essential part of any system of healthcare, to pick up poor care or obsolete standards and to promote higher ones. In parallel, each specialty and subspecialty should ideally have at least one activist patient group studying it, rather as political parties out of power shadow those in power (Williamson, 2000a). To some extent, single-disease or condition patient groups do this. But how effective and how radical they are varies (Chapter Eight).

◊◊ In 1990, I asked a doctor-dominated charity for heart disease if it were aware that admission to some coronary care units was barred to patients over a certain age. Yes, it was aware. But it refused to give me the names of any units that had, or did not have, the ban. ◊◊

In the past, from 1948 to the 1980s, new policies that potentially harmed patients' interests were usually devised and introduced by professionals. Now corporate rationalisers play a significant part in setting standards of care, although professionals still have the power to refuse to implement them (Chapter Two). But patient activists have not given enough attention to corporate rationalism to be able to analyse its effects on patients' interests. They need to do this urgently.

◊◊ Some primary care trusts, for example, Oxfordshire Primary Care Trust, pay GPs to reduce the numbers of patients they refer to hospital specialists (Moore and Roland, 2008). Giving financial incentives (bribes) to GPs to do something so potentially harmful to patients' interests should have been opposed. But the decision was taken without patients and the public being told about it in advance or being able to comment on it. ◊◊

Conclusions

Some of the principles that radical patient activism has promoted have been espoused by other parts of the patient movement and by patients, although it is difficult to say exactly who has adopted what, when and from where. The principles have spread to health professionals and to corporate rationalisers, though putting them into practice through standards of care is problematic. The rhetoric is on the right lines, but the train easily gets derailed.

Some specific changes to standards of care can be attributed to radical patient activists' initiatives and persistence. (There are examples in Chapters Four and Five, as well in this chapter.) Patients probably now take these standards for granted or expect them to prevail when they experience healthcare. To that extent, radical ideas have spread and become accepted by 'ordinary' patients. But some old issues remain unresolved and some regression has taken place.

As healthcare changes, patient activists will identify new issues. Much remains for radical patient activists to do, both now and as new practices and standards are introduced. But radical patient activism has had some success in emancipating patients from some aspects of coercion in healthcare.

ELEVEN

What next?

If the patient movement is not an emancipation movement, what is it?

(Andrew Smith, anaesthetist, 2009, personal communication)

Introduction

Radical patient activists have established the principles they wish to see expressed through the values given to standards of treatment and care. In Chapter Six I noted that two basic principles of recognised emancipation movements, *justice* and *equality*, have not been adopted as principles by radical patient activists. In this chapter, I show that they are already implicit in radical patient activism's principles. I suggest that it is time they were made explicit. That would flag up radical patient activism, and hence the patient movement, as an emancipation movement. That could be scary, for emancipation movements arouse hostility at first. But three benefits could follow: it could make sense of the patient side of healthcare; it could help make healthcare worthy of the aspirations of those who give it; and it could give us new theoretical underpinnings for improving some aspects of the quality of healthcare.

Justice

Justice has a strong moral appeal. Doing morally right was an early meaning of justice, and although that meaning is now archaic, the word 'just' still means morally right, fair, equitable, giving everyone their due, what is fair and right for all people (Little et al, 1936; Brown, 1993). Justice is a principle of the women's, the black liberation, the disability rights and the civil rights movements (Miles, 1988; Groch, 2001; Kemper, 2001). Other smaller movements have also adopted it. Homosexual activists, for example, press for justice and equal rights to medical care for homosexuals, and animal rights activists advocate justice for animals (Gould, 2001; Groves, 2001). Western legal systems are, in part, a means for protecting weaker individuals against more powerful ones (Annas, 1975). Rights movements and emancipation movements try to get some policies, practices and standards enshrined as legally enforceable rights, as conditions that must always be met (Annas, 1975). Aspirational 'rights' can sometimes be changed into legal rights through court action, which sometimes favours the less powerful person or group (Annas, 1975). Both legal and aspirational rights are covered by the concept of justice.

Justice is not an explicit principle of radical patient activism, but it is implicit in six of its explicit principles:

1. **Respect for patients' autonomy**, for their personhoods, is fundamental to justice. Power is exercised *unjustly* if it impairs people's ability to develop and exercise their capabilities as individual people, communicating and cooperating with others (Young, 1990; Chapter Two). Impairing, inhibiting or preventing patients from acting, within the law, autonomously and as moral agents, is unjust. Radical patient activism's emphasis on patient autonomy and its opposition to coercion constitute its most cogent support for the principle of *justice*.

2. **Equity**, especially equity as levelling up. Here, *justice* as fairness between patients, making available to all patients the opportunities and benefits that some patients can have, comes in.

3. **Access** for all patients to the services, the information, and so on, that might help them, is close kin to equity (Chapter Seven); fairness and *justice* come in here.

4. **Redress** is concerned with *justice* in its basic legal sense. Justice for patients must be patient activism's primary objective. But that includes justice for staff, because only rigorous, impartial and independent examination of evidence can secure justice for patients (Chapter Seven).

   Making other systems fairer to patients also comes under redress.

   ◊◊ The Patient Liaison Group of the Royal College of General Practitioners' guidance to GPs, telling them that they must warn patients that they might be struck off the practice list, and should give them reasons and an opportunity to discuss the matter with the GP (Chapter Nine), is an example of giving information to patients in order to make the system *less unjust*, as well as of trying to change professional practice. ◊◊

5. **Safety** is partly concerned with justice because unsafe practices usually put patients at greater risk of danger than they put staff (Chapter Seven). This is *unjust* as between patients and staff. It is

a good example of how the repression of patients' interests and injustice towards them are closely linked

6. **Information includes trying to ensure that professionals and corporate rationalisers do not act secretly**. Secrecy often surrounds three major sorts of professionals' and corporate rationalisers' actions. Those actions may include secrecies to do with rationing, with clinical decisions unrelated to rationing and with staff's preferences or convenience.

Rationing

The government and the medical profession have a contract whereby doctors engage in rationing healthcare inconspicuously and without necessarily telling their patients that they are denying something that could benefit them (New and Le Grand, 1996). Secrecy about rationing is *unjust* because it means that patients are, in effect, on trial in the GP's surgery or the hospital, without knowing that they are on trial and with no opportunity to defend their own interests or to contest the decision. Some patients are aware that doctors ration care, but they hope that their doctor will not jeopardise their welfare (Mechanic, 2004). This is not an endorsement of rationing, however, for to endorse rationing one would have to be willing to be harmed or deprived oneself.

The larger issue of whether rationing is or is not necessary in rich western countries is not immediately relevant here. Here the issues are: who decides what shall be rationed; how it is carried out; whether and how individual patients should be told that their treatment and care will be, or will not be, restricted in some way, and why; and how they can appeal against a local decision or go elsewhere for treatment (Williamson, 2005).

The profession's belief that it must act for the common good of patients, for populations of patients, as well as for individual patients, is a belief not wrong in itself. Patients, too, want to see resources used wisely and for the benefit of all (Coulter, 2005). But this belief perhaps blinds doctors to the gravity and to the *injustice* of rationing done secretly, without the knowledge of the patients who are affected by it. Or doctors may feel that they are merely carrying out the government's and corporate rationalisers' wishes and requirements, and so need feel no personal responsibility for harm to patients.

◊◊ "Why should we do the government's dirty work for it?" said a medically qualified chief executive of a trust, meaning that the government, not the hospital, should tell patients which drugs they could not have in that hospital (personal observation, 1997). ◊◊

This view, however, is morally questionable in a profession that wants patients to trust it.

Power to make other decisions

Individual clinicians, or teams of professionals, have extraordinary power to make decisions about what treatment and care will be, or will not be, offered to patients, even when they are not rationing treatments because of their expense.

> ◊◊ A National Confidential Enquiry into Patient Outcome and Death [NCEPOD] publication describes good practice as follows. Whether patients with advanced cancer should be offered systemic anti-cancer therapy is decided at a team meeting at which the patient is neither present nor represented. If the team decides to offer therapy, the patient is fully informed about its possible benefits and risks and can decide whether to accept or decline it (NCEPOD, 2008). ◊◊

This policy is well meant, since these patients are very ill and may have little hope of surviving, whatever is done, and the therapies can be harsh and dangerous. But it misses out what some people would see as the most crucial stage at which the patient should be present, or represented, if he or she wishes, the first stage. If the team decides to offer therapy, no harm is done. But if it decides not to offer therapy, the patient is denied knowledge of that stage and of participation in it. It is a mark of the power of dominant interest holders that this example can be taken from an official publication, where the policy above is recommended without any awareness of its *injustice*.

Staff preferences and convenience

Policies may be concealed from patients so as to meet the personal preferences or convenience of staff (Williamson, 2005). This again prevents patients from speaking for their views and interests, and again, is *unjust*.

Chapter Ten gave examples in maternity care where midwives did not offer the national MIDIRS leaflets to women. Here, research and patients' accounts of their experiences reveal matters that the profession itself would probably regard as disturbing. That these practices can continue to occur, though, is again a mark of the repression of patients' interests and of the freedom of dominant interest holders to act as they choose.

Equality

Equality means having equal or the same status, power, esteem or other good as other people or groups (Brown, 1993). Equality has a fundamental ethical, social and political appeal in western democratic countries. Equality is a principle of emancipation movements like the black civil rights and the women's movements (Franklin, 1947; Miles, 1988). Again, it is not an explicit principle of radical patient activism.

Equality's strong appeal is hard to reconcile with reality in hierarchical or socially stratified societies. In practice, democratic equality may come down to equality of voice through the ballot box and equality before the law. But equality with other social groups is a powerful aspiration for weaker groups. For weaker groups to seek equality is a politically apt strategic approach to a strong group that can coerce or oppress its members, but whose goodwill and skills they need (Williamson, 2008a). Exactly what is meant by equality in healthcare is difficult to define. Patients who are sick or disabled have some physiological, biochemical or anatomical differences from people who are well. These are biological differences, not merely socially constructed ones. A society might choose to invest sick people with glory instead of with disadvantage. But that would not stop them dying of their diseases, unless they were treated effectively. These biological differences are like those between males and females that lead to the equality/difference debates among feminists (Freedman, 2001). In what senses can people who are evidently different in physical strength and capability and in physical vulnerability at some stages of their lives be equal to people who are not? What of our evolutionary heritage (Chapter Two)?

For patients, *equality* of moral agency; *equality* of voice; and *equality* of respect and esteem, recognition of full status as a human being, seem to be what matter most. Patients' wish to be treated 'as people', 'as a person', shows their wish for equality with health professionals, for no one supposes that professionals are not people. It is equality with members of the relevant dominant group or groups that is sought, blacks with whites, disabled people with able-bodied people. It is not universal equality, a more ambitious objective.

Although equality is not an explicit principle for radical patient activism, it is implicit in four of its principles:

1. **Shared decision making** encompasses equality of moral agency with clinicians through *equality of voice* in the individual patient–clinician relationship.

   ◊◊ The Insulin Dependent Diabetic Trust declares that 'patient views [should] carry equal weight [with clinicians] in decision making about their treatment' (IDDT, 2006). ◊◊

   Equality of voice is linked to power.

   ◊◊ 'Power is the ability to take one's place in whatever discourse is essential to action and the right to have one's part matter.' (Heilbrun, 1989, p 18) ◊◊

2. **Choice** within the law is one of the conditions people draw on to express their autonomy and to direct the purposes of their lives (Chapter Seven). Choice is linked both to access and to freedom from the injustices, coercions and *inequalities* that inhibit people from making autonomous choices.

3. **Support**. Patients sometimes need a relative or friend or professional advocate with them in consultations with clinicians, in order to hold them up emotionally in difficult discussions, to strengthen their voice and to ensure that the clinician understands their wishes.

   ◊◊ A patient who had had two courses of chemotherapy for advanced cancer asked for a third course. His oncologist demurred, on the grounds that it would almost certainly be ineffective. The patient's wife successfully pressed for the third course. It was ineffective and the patient stopped it. But the oncologist later said that he hoped, were he seriously ill, to have someone as articulate and determined as the wife had been to speak for him (Graeme Moodie, personal communication, 2007). ◊◊

   Ensuring that patients can have support, when they wish, respects their *equality of moral agency* with the clinician's own.

4. **Representation**. The patient movement, not just radical patient activists, wants to see *equality of voice* between patients and doctors collectively, and between patients and corporate rationalisers collectively, in policy making at every level of the health service. This raises issues about representation (Chapter Seven). These issues

apply to all interest holders, for example, to nurses, not just to patients. The diversity of patients and the repression of their interests, however, probably makes speaking for their interests more difficult and problematic than speaking for those of doctors or nurses or physiotherapists, either in general or over specific issues. For one thing, the factions in the patient movement are probably less readily recognised than are those between and among different groups of health professionals.

◊◊ Differences between anaesthetists and surgeons in their approaches to the same patients are recognised and understood (Fox, 1992). Differences between radical and conservative patient groups' or individual activists' approaches to the standards of care that they would like to see in place are not so well recognised (Chapter Eight). ◊◊

In spite of difficulties, equality of voice in representation must always fundamentally be about equality of power, of power shared equally. Equality of voice expresses equality of power where it matters most to patients, in collective and individual decisions about their, their families' and their community's healthcare. But only through equality of power can equality of voice be guaranteed.

Recognising the patient movement as an emancipation movement

Once a social movement has come to see that its aim is equality of power between its social group and the more powerful social group or groups denying it that equality, it has become an emancipation movement. It would be risky, however, for the patient movement to declare itself an emancipation movement. It would arouse increased misunderstanding and hostility. But there could be at least three gains. First, people could think more clearly about the social group to be emancipated. Second, dominant interest holders could see that in some ways emancipation could benefit them, both by making their care worthy of their moral and ethical aspirations and in practical ways. Third, it could work towards improving the quality of care in the health service.

Patients as a social group: making sense of the patient side of healthcare

Health professionals, corporate rationalisers, lay people and patients themselves can be confused or uncertain about who are 'patients', how to find out what they think, and who can speak about their experiences or speak for their interests (Chapters Seven and Nine).

◊◊ A survey company, commissioned to find out patients' views on blood transfusion, took samples of patients from several out-patients' departments. It did not try to sample patients who had had a blood transfusion or who expected to have one (personal observation, 1997). ◊◊

In recognised emancipation movements, all the people in the social group for whom emancipation is sought are regarded as members of that social group: all women, all black people in a country whose dominant population is white, all homosexuals. People who do not regard themselves as members of a movement ("I'm not a feminist") or who take no part in its work are regarded as non-activist or 'ordinary' members (Chapter Nine). Attributing notional membership to people who would reject it is high-handed. But non-activists are extremely important as part of the movement's matrix, the social conditions from which it springs and which sustain it.

Non-activists

1. It is from non-activists that activists often pick up and explore fresh insights and new perceptions (Chapter Five).

2. There are always fewer activists than non-activists. It is non-activists who select and adapt activists' ideas and spread them to each other, to professionals and through society in general (Mansbridge, 2001a; Chapter Ten). The non-activists select ideas that appeal to them, probably often those that support their autonomy, even if they do not consciously recognise why those ideas appeal to them.

◊◊ The simple message of NAWCH, your child in hospital needs you, you should not be prevented from being there, appealed to the mothers of young children. Some mothers may have recognised intuitively the link to autonomy, though probably not all. But taking personal or group action can appeal to people's sense of their own autonomy and efficacy as well as to their social conscience. ◊◊

3. Non-activists can spread ideas or higher standards just by asking for something. Professionals' and corporate rationalisers' prejudices against patient activists can make the requests of 'ordinary' or 'real' patients convincing, even if activists have already argued the same case in vain.

> ◊ ◊ A non-activist patient who asks for something he or she has heard or read about that is not normally offered or permitted in a particular hospital or GP practice can change professionals' ideas and set a precedent for other patients. There is always a successful first: a woman who asks to have her husband present at the birth of their baby; a patient scheduled for elective surgery who asks for an autologous blood transfusion. ◊◊

4. Activists are recruited from non-activists. They start new activist groups or join old ones.

> ◊ ◊ The talks NAWCH activist members gave in the 1960s to women's and community groups, 'ordinary' parents, moved many young mothers to join NAWCH (Chapter Five). ◊◊

5. Non-activists' expectations and criticisms of care can show the extent to which activists' ideas have been accepted by society and its 'ordinary' members (Chapter Ten).

Once non-activists have been separated conceptually from activists, we can begin to see how each plays their part in healthcare and its politics. We know that non-activist patients differ from each other in how much information, shared decision making, and so on, they want, and what they take these terms to mean (Edwards and Elwyn, 2006; Chapter Seven). Activists, too, differ in regular ways from each other, with the distinction between radical and conservative activists being especially important (Chapters Eight and Nine). Once these distinctions can be made, we can get a clearer view of some of the aspects of the patient side of healthcare that can seem confusing.

> ◊ ◊ Many aspects of healthcare are "like a jigsaw puzzle in which some of the pieces are missing and from which people are always picking up the wrong pieces" (Nancy Hill, non-executive director

of Leeds Northwest Primary Care Trust, personal communication, 2004). ◊◊

Supplying some of the missing pieces can help people to pick up the right ones.

Making healthcare worthy of the aspirations of those who give it

On becoming patients, people enter a world that neither they nor the people who went before them into that world took part in forming. They become subject to policies and practices of which they knew nothing. They take parts in plays whose script they had no part in writing. The conditions imposed upon them may benefit or threaten their interests, as they would define their interests, were they aware of the possible benefits and the possible threats (Chapter Two). Patients' exclusion from setting the conditions that concern them so fundamentally makes it unsurprising that they can be subject to coercions, injustices and inequalities: their interests have been so thoroughly repressed.

Yet at the same time, the health professionals and corporate rationalisers who are the instruments of coercions, injustices and inequalities may be unaware of how their actions affect patients and patients' interests (Chapter Two). For healthcare, a deeply moral enterprise, this is tragic. Professionals' good intentions deserve to be held in honour. But they are not enough: good intentions can be too remote from the effects of the actions or the inactions that they prompt.

It is here that the patient movement as an emancipation movement, examining the effects of professionals' and corporate rationalisers' actions upon patients (Chapter Five), can help these dominant interest holders to meet their own aspirations. This is perhaps most obvious in patient activists' detailed work in trying to improve specific standards of care. There they raise their own and professionals' consciousness about current standards and support that consciousness with evidence and argument. Activists' concern is for patients; but lessening oppression relieves the oppressors of the unease, even guilt, that they may come to feel once their consciousness has been raised. So when activists succeed, professionals' opposition can turn into gratitude: sometimes activists have made things better, not worse, for them as well as for patients.

◊◊ Welcoming parents into paediatric wards keeps children calmer and lets parents carry out some tasks for their children, freeing nurses for other tasks. Nurses have no cause to feel guilt about separating children from their parents and are not exposed to parents' anger at being excluded from the ward. ◊◊

◊◊ It took six years to get narrow windows, high up in the walls of the labour rooms in the maternity unit of a hospital replaced by ordinary-sized windows, at a level at which the room's occupants could see out, rather than being imprisoned in an unpleasant and unnatural space. Managers allocated the money. But midwives repeatedly opposed the change. Eventually, the issue was raised at the (governance) board, who agreed that patients should be cared for in environments conducive to their comfort. After the windows were altered, the midwives sent word that they, as well as women in labour, liked the new windows; they improved their working environment (Williamson, 1994). ◊◊

Improving the quality of healthcare

The quality of healthcare is of constant concern both to the providers and to the recipients of that healthcare in the UK, the US and other western countries. Experts, commentators and documents are plentiful. New ideas and schemes arise, have their moments of promise and hope, and fall back into oblivion. Can the ethical and moral force and the ideas of emancipation do better? Emancipation movements look beyond the particular social groups with which they are concerned, to the values and hopes of wider society. They look to humanity itself. The assumptions and biases of any one social group should be subordinate to those wider, more abstract values. Here these values include justice and equality.

Justice and equality are inspiring ideas. Putting them into operation requires sensitivity, thought and political skill, attributes that many professionals and corporate rationalisers have. Every policy, practice and standard, every familiar way of doing things, or proposed new way, should be considered in the light of justice and equality. Justice and equality are not relevant to all standards. But for others, they could provide the theoretical underpinning that could lead to improved quality, higher standards.

◊◊ After a patient has seen a hospital specialist, some specialists write only to the patient's GP, others send the patient a copy of that letter (Chapter Ten). Addressing the letter to both the patient and the GP would symbolise equality between all three. ◊◊

That same policy, practice or standard could be promoted under the rubrics of *information, respect, safety* or *shared decision making*. But equality is a more absolute principle. It indicates what course of action should be taken, more clearly and more cogently. Small symbolic actions like this can alter the ways people feel and think about and so relate to each other. Individuals' actions can, collectively and eventually, result in structural changes to society. Recognised emancipation movements show us that.

The example just given illustrates equality of esteem. Equality of voice also matters (Chapter Seven). Equality of voice in healthcare points to the importance of all three major social groups of interest holders being represented at every discussion that could affect the interests of any of them. Each group's representatives should analyse its group's interests and explain them to the other interest holders clearly and truthfully. This they ought to do at all times, for ethics consists of searching for the best way to harmonise groups' or individuals' interests with those of others (Tong, 1997). But most particularly, they ought to do it whenever current standards of care are reviewed or new ones are proposed. Thorough discussion of the interests of each group would sometimes reveal irreconcilable conflicts of those interests. Then the most powerful group or groups of interest holders would prevail, just as they do now. At other times, the different interest holders could arrive at courses of action, new policies, practices or standards, that met the purposes of each while preserving each's own perspective and definition of their interests (Chapter Nine). To work towards equality between dominant and subordinate groups, it is the subordinate group that must define its own interests and the dominant groups that must take them into account in their own actions (Chapter Nine).

◊ ◊ Corporate rationalisers introduced a system in 2006 for managing (controlling) GPs' referrals of patients to specialists. GPs' letters of referral are diverted to referral centres, where they are forwarded to a specialist, referred to another kind of health professional or barred (Davies and Elwyn, 2006). Corporate rationalisers intend to make referrals more appropriate, as judged by the referral centre; to get data on each GP's referrals to check against trusts' claims for payment; to see whether GPs are complying with referral guidelines; and to gain more control over GPs by edging out their clinical autonomy (Williamson, 2008b). As a side effect, referral management reduces patients' autonomy. That is because a decision to refer a patient is, or should be, a shared decision between the patient and the GP.

With referral management, a third party enters the relationship. Some GPs opposed referral management because of the threat to their autonomy, but failed to halt it (Williamson, 2008b). Questions about patients' autonomy; about the reviewers' access to the patients' medical records; about patients' rights of appeal against barred or delayed referrals, seem to have been unasked (Williamson, 2008b). Not asking questions, here rather obvious ones, is an aspect of repression. Nor does referral management help patients' worries that their GPs may fail to refer them when they should. Patients and patient representatives were not invited to take part in discussions between clinicians and corporate rationalisers about this major change to healthcare in the UK. ◊◊

Yet had patients and patient representatives taken part, other ways of securing 'better' referrals probably could have been found. For example, if patients were routinely offered the referral guidelines for the disease or disorder they or they GP suspected, the patient and GP could go through the guidelines together and discuss whether they should be followed, in the light of the patient's predicament, and any other information or views the patient and the GP might have. That would protect the patient's safety. It would respect the autonomy of both patient and GP. GPs would become accustomed to following referral guidelines, unless there were a reason not to. This would meet corporate rationalisers' interests in securing cost-effective, adequate standards of care for populations of patients. The repression of patients' interests both through some GPs' inattention to guidelines and through the current referral management scheme could have been avoided (Williamson, 2008b).

Acting in the light of equality of voice can raise standards of healthcare. Men collectively have benefited from the women's movement and white people from the black civil rights movement. Emancipation sets people free to contribute creatively and imaginatively to society. At the same time, emancipation movements point to the importance of members of subordinate social groups educating themselves and showing that they are competent to play a part equal to that of dominant interest holders.

◊◊ Coaching patients before consultations can enable them and their clinicians to share their knowledge and insights with each other more freely. In one study, some patients were briefed with a booklet and a video about clinical decision making for breast cancer, other patients were not so briefed (Rhoda Brown et al,

2004). Oncologists talked more with the patients who had been briefed than with the unbriefed control group. Not only did the oncologists respond more fully to topics that the briefed patients raised, they also raised more new topics themselves (Rhoda Brown et al, 2004). ◊◊

This suggests that some clinicians would find consultations to which patients could contribute their knowledge and ideas more rewarding than those to which patients could contribute little. Not all patients want to spend time and effort on thinking about their own clinical condition, or about issues for patients collectively or about healthcare politics. But we know from recognised emancipation movements that not all need to; a few can change dominant interest holders' assumptions and behaviours.

Perhaps the most important aspect of equality is equality of moral agency. Some clinicians seem to deny moral agency to patients (Chapters One and Four). Or they decide that patients' actions show that patients lack proper moral standards. Emancipation movements' experience suggests that members of dominant groups are apt to attribute derogatory traits and characteristics to subordinate groups (Chapter One). Do some clinicians and some corporate rationalisers do the same? Do they tend to put denigratory interpretations on patients' actions? Do clinicians and managers in some fundamental, but probably not wholly conscious, sense tend to see patients collectively as stupid or selfish or irresponsible?

◊◊ A doctor in training to become a consultant recently wrote that patients who asked to see the consultant at an out-patient clinic, instead of accepting whichever trainee doctor they had been allocated to, were probably 'assertive patients attempting to gain an unfair advantage' over other patients (Crampsey, 2009, p 955). '[These patients' actions are] both ethically and morally questionable' (Crampsey, 2009, p 955). This doctor sees such requests, moreover, as an insult to all doctors in training and a challenge to himself. He believes that such requests should be refused (Crampsey, 2009). ◊◊

From patients' points of view, out-patient clinics are often ill-managed. Patients are seldom told anything about the doctors present in the clinic, whether they are clinical assistants or doctors in training, for example, and if the latter, at what stage of their training they are. Patients returning to a clinic because of chronic or recurrent diseases or for routine follow-up are not usually invited to say whether they particularly want to see the consultant this time or would be happy with another doctor. The consultant responsible for their care has the necessary knowledge, experience and skill to take that responsibility; and patients can build up over time a good relationship with him or her. But doctors in training can be easier to talk to and sometimes impart extra information or explanation. Some patients would be happy to see a doctor in training sometimes, provided that they knew that if they or the trainee doctor felt any doubt during the consultation, they could ask the consultant to join them. Yet to find out whom they are going to see, patients usually have to wait until they are summoned into a consulting room. The uncertainty and suspense of these arrangements is discourteous to patients as well as hard on those patients who particularly hoped to see the consultant this time. In a flawed system like this, patients are more likely to be trying to protect their own health (a legitimate objective in a healthcare institution) than to do down each other.

Some health professionals' readiness to attribute low moral status to patients is relevant to quality and standards because health professionals' negative attributions and interpretations may lead them to tolerate poor standards of care. Low standards of care and failures by doctors or nurses to treat patients as people are usually explained by too few staff, too few resources, stressful working environments (Goodrich and Cornwell, 2008). These play a part. But emancipation movements point to the likelihood of other, less easily remedied factors, deeper cultural and institutionalised feelings. If dominant interest holders hold a negative view of subordinate interest holders, there are likely to be harmful consequences for staff as well as for patients. Too few staff, poorly trained staff or staff lacking adequate support or pleasant working conditions reflect the repression of patients' interests through the financial arrangements for the health service and the political decisions about how much money should be spent and by whom. The primary responsibility for inadequate or poorly allocated resources lies with corporate rationalisers and the official agencies whom they serve. To a large extent, however, health professionals' acceptance of a make-do-and-mend approach to better facilities, more staff, better training, more time for consultations, more effective diagnostic tests and treatments, has acted against patients' interests as well as against professionals' own interests. If clinicians and corporate rationalisers could recognise the part that their own negative attributions and assumptions about patients probably play in sustaining low standards of care, it would be possible to raise standards and avoid some of the worst practices so evident in healthcare today. If they could see how the repression of patients' interests has pervasive ill consequences, they could start to lift that repression in a host of minor and major ways.

Last words

Patient activists have to work by persuasion and influence. To do that, they have to affect the moral and ethical sensibilities of professionals and corporate rationalisers so that they no longer accept some policies, practices and standards. Some of today's standards should be as inconceivable tomorrow as slavery or women's disenfranchisement are today. Different emancipation movements confront different issues; but the changes in moral and ethical sensibility required in order to lift repression and oppression are the same.

In spite of the benefits of emancipation to the other interest holders, as well as to subordinate social groups, emancipation is a long and hard journey. Recognised emancipation movements show us this. So do the last 50 years of radical patient activism in western countries. But it is a journey with hope, the hope of making healthcare better for everyone.

> ... *concern about goodness, rightness and justness ... has a powerful presence – manifest or latent – in our minds.*
>
> (Amartya Sen, 2009, p 414)

The principal component analysis

Community health councils' (CHCs) annual reports were their public statements about themselves, their activities and their achievements. They were also public statements of the CHCs' positions on controversial issues. In the 45 annual reports, as noted in Chapter Eight, I found about 46 pairs of incompatible positions, for example, whether or not patients should have access to their medical notes or whether or not members of the public should be allowed to speak at CHC meetings. Of these 46 pairs, I found 10 pairs of incompatible positions, one or other of which was recorded in all 45 annual reports. Some were matters of fact: the CHC office either was or was not on the premises of a hospital. Some were statements of aim or belief. Some were positive or negative judgements: 'the CHC observer at the Area Health Authority meeting expressed concern at the inadequate knowledge she felt had been displayed by the members of the Authority [the non-executive directors], and at the low standard of debate at the Authority's meetings'.

The 10 pairs of incompatible positions meant almost nothing to me, beyond their face value. As different mixes of the 10 incompatible positions held by each CHC, they made no sense at all. So principal component analysis (PCA) was a good exploratory technique for seeing whether there were a hidden basis or bases for the conflicts that could be observed in some CHCs, conflicts that were presumably reflected or indicated by their incompatible positions on the 10 issues. I scored each indicator position as +1 or −1 consistently within each pair of positions, but at random in relation to all the other nine pairs. That is, the incompatible positions could be regarded as dichotomous variables with reversible polarities, just as hot/cold is the same as not cold/not hot. That was a requirement of the method, to avoid scoring in spurious relationships (correlations). PCA examines the mathematical structure of data, not their meanings. It enables hidden aspects of data to be seen and it makes no assumptions about the probability distribution of the original variables, here the incompatible positions (Chatfield and Collins, 1980). So it is not like looking for correlations between variables whose meaning is known. That is why it does not matter whether positions are scored as plus or as minus, as long as it is done consistently for each pair of incompatible positions for all 45 CHCs. Mark Williamson designed and carried out the principal component analysis of the 45 × 10 matrix of these plus and minus scores.

Figure A.1: The 45 community health councils' scores

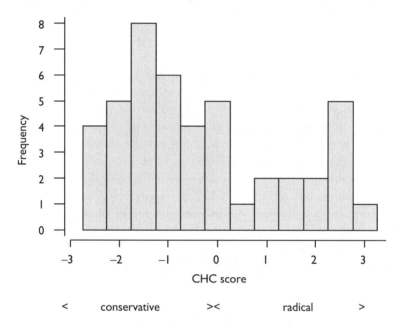

The result is described in Chapter Eight. The analysis produced a new bipolar variable, the first principal component, with high plus scores at one end and high minus scores at the other. Most CHCs held a mix of incompatible positions, some positions with high loadings on the first principal component, others with low loadings. Where pluses and minuses cancelled each other out, the score was zero, the mathematical point that divided CHCs into plus CHCs or minus CHCs. The first principal component accounted for almost 30% of the variance, roughly twice as much as that accounted for by the second principal component. Thirty per cent did not look like very much; but the test here was whether meanings could be attributed to the principal components that were consonant with other, independent variables. A few of the variables significantly associated with CHCs' scores for the first principal component were noted in Chapter Eight. (Others, to do with other parts of the research, are discussed in my thesis, Williamson, 1983). The meaning I gave to the first principal component is explained in Chapter Eight. I thought the second and third might be frugality versus extravagance and connectedness versus isolation. They were unimportant for my purposes, but they are a reminder that people and groups almost always act from more than one motive.

The difficulty of this method was in finding enough incompatible positions to score, and hoping that some of them were important enough as causes of conflict within and between CHCs to make what they meant matter theoretically. Some positions had only one indicator, but others had two or three that I assumed stood for the same position. Putting them together as one position does not bias the analysis if the indicators are apt. If they are not apt, it reduces the clarity of the results by introducing random error, but does not distort them. Very rarely, an annual report contained indicators for both incompatible positions. Then I took the one with greater emphasis or the more negative expression, since adverse comments are usually more salient than favourable comments.

References

Note: For some sorts of writing, a patient's accounts of his or her care, for example, it can be useful to know the author's gender. I have therefore included authors' first names whenever possible.

Abel-Smith, Brian (1964) *The hospitals 1800–1948: A study in social administration*, London: Heinemann.

AIMS (Association for Improvements in the Maternity Services) and NCT (National Childbirth Trust) (1997) *A charter for ethical research in maternity care*, London: AIMS and NCT.

Alderson, Priscilla, Hawthorne, Joanna and Killen, Margaret (2005) 'The participation rights of premature babies', *The International Journal of Children's Rights*, vol 13, pp 31–50.

Alderson, Priscilla, Hawthorne, Joanna and Killen, Margaret (2006) 'Parents' experiences of sharing neonatal information and decisions: Consent, cost and risk', *Social Science & Medicine*, vol 62, pp 1319–29.

Alderson, Priscilla, Madden, Mary, Oakley, Ann and Wilkins, Ruth (1994) *Women's views of breast cancer treatment and research, Report of a pilot project 1993*, London: Social Science Research Unit, Institute of Education, University of London.

Alford, Robert R. (1975) *Health care politics: Ideological and interest group barriers to reform*, Chicago: University of Chicago Press.

Allsop, Judith and Mulcahy, Linda (1999) 'Doctors' responses to patient complaints', in Marilynn M. Rosenthal, Linda Mulcahy and Sally Lloyd-Bostock (eds) *Medical mishaps: Pieces of the puzzle*, Buckingham: Open University Press, pp 124–40.

Allsop, Judith, Jones, Kathryn and Baggott, Rob (2004) 'Health consumer groups in the UK: a new social movement?', *Sociology of Health & Illness*, vol 26, no 6, pp 737–56.

Andrea (2001) 'Father as witness', Letter to *Midwifery Matters*, vol 88, Spring, p 33.

Annas, George J. (1975) *The rights of hospital patients: The basic ACLU [American Civil Liberties Union] guide to a hospital patient's rights*, New York: Avon Books.

Annas, George J. (1998) 'A national bill of patients' rights', *New England Journal of Medicine*, vol 338, no 10, pp 695–9.

Anon (1982) 'Human relations in obstetrics: Father knows best?' *AIMS Quarterly Journal*, Spring, pp 1–3.

Anon (1998) 'The ostrich view of the world', *The Economist*, vol 349, p 39.

Anon (2007/8) 'Informed consent', *AIMS Journal*, vol 19, no 4, pp 10–11.

Arksey, Hilary (1994) 'Expert and lay participation in the construction of medical knowledge', *Sociology of Health & Illness*, vol 16, no 4, pp 448–68.

Armstrong, David and Ogden, Jane (2006) 'The role of etiquette and experimentation in explaining how doctors change behaviour: A qualitative study', *Sociology of Health & Illness*, vol 28, no 7, pp 951–68.

Armstrong, S[arah] L. (2009) 'A view from the other end of the laryngoscope', *Bulletin of the Royal College of Anaesthetists*, vol 54, pp 39–41.

Austoker, Joan, Mansel, Robert, Baum, Michael, Sainsbury, Richard and Hobbs, Richard (1995) *Guidelines for referral of patients with breast problems*, Sheffield: NHS Breast Screening Programme.

Baggott, Rob, Allsop, Judith and Jones, Kathryn (2005) *Speaking for patients and carers: Health consumer groups and the policy process*, Basingstoke: Palgrave Macmillan.

Bate, Paul and Robert, Glenn (2007) *Bringing user experience to healthcare improvement: The concepts, methods and practices of experience-based design*, Oxford: Radcliffe Publishing.

Bate, P[aul], Robert, G[lenn] and Bevan, H. (2004) 'The next phase of healthcare improvement: what can we learn from social movements?', *Quality & Safety in Health Care*, vol 13, pp 62–6.

Bates, Claire (2001) 'The good doctor', *Clinical Medicine*, vol 1, no 2, pp 128–31.

Bates, Thelma and Evans, Richard G.B. (1995) *Report of the independent review commissioned by the Royal College of Radiologists into brachial plexus neuropathy following radiotherapy for breast carcinoma*, London: Royal College of Radiologists.

Batt, Sharon (1994) *Patient no more: The politics of breast cancer*, London: Scarlet Press.

Beech, Beverley (2004/5) 'Episiotomy: Still a sore subject', *AIMS Journal*, vol 16, no 4, pp 18–19.

Beech, Beverley (2005) 'Choice – an abused concept that is past its sell-by date', *AIMS Journal*, vol 17, no 4, pp 3–4.

Belson, Peg (1981) 'Parents' advocacy for parents', in Pat Azarnoff and Carol Hardgrove (eds) *The family in child health care*, New York: John Wiley & Sons, pp 217–31.

Belson, Peg (2004) 'To get our agenda on other people's agenda', in Helene Curtis and Mimi Sanderson (eds), *The unsung sixties: Memoirs of social innovation*, London: Whiting & Birch Ltd, pp 357–70.

Berwick, Donald M. (2003) 'Errors today and errors tomorrow', *New England Journal of Medicine*, vol 348, no 25, pp 2570–2.

Bewley, Susan (1992) 'The law, medical students and assault', *BMJ*, vol 304, pp 1551–3,

Birkinshaw, Patrick (1994) *Grievances, remedies and the state* (2nd edn), London: Sweet & Maxwell.

Blenkinsopp, A[lison], Wilkie, P[atricia], Wang, M[adeleine] and Routledge, P[hilip] A. (2006) 'Patient reporting of suspected adverse drug reactions: a review of published literature and international experience', *British Journal of Clinical Pharmacology*, vol 63, no 2, pp 148–56.

Blennerhassett, Mitzi (1998) 'Truth, the first casualty', *BMJ*, vol 316, pp 1890–1.

Blennerhassett, Mitzi (2008) *Nothing personal: Disturbing undercurrents in cancer care*, Oxford: Radcliff Publishing.

Borkman, Thomasina (1997) 'A selective look at self-help groups in the United States', *Health and Social Care in the Community*, vol 5, no 6, pp 357–64.

Bosk, Charles L. (1979) *Forgive and remember: Managing medical failure*, Chicago: University of Chicago Press.

Bourdieu, Pierre (1998) *Practical reason: On the theory of action*, Cambridge: Polity Press.

Bowlby, John (1965) *Child care and the growth of love* (2nd edn), Harmondsworth: Penguin Books, abridged from *Maternal care and mental health* (1951), Geneva: World Health Organisation.

Brain, D.J. and Maclay, Inga (1968) 'Controlled study of mothers and children in hospital', *BMJ*, vol 2, pp 278–80.

Bristol Royal Infirmary Inquiry (2000) *Interim report, Removal and retention of human material, Annex A*. London: Central Office of Information.

Bristol Royal Infirmary Inquiry (2001) *Learning from Bristol: The report of the public inquiry into children's heart surgery at the Bristol Royal Infirmary, 1984–1995*, London: Stationery Office.

British Geriatric Society and Royal College of Nursing (1975) *Improving geriatric care in hospital*, London: Royal College of Nursing.

British Medical Association, Resuscitation Council (UK) and Royal College of Nursing (2001) *Decisions relating to cardiopulmonary resuscitation*, London: British Medical Council.

British Medical Association and Royal Pharmaceutical Society of Great Britain (2004) *British national formulary*, London: British Medical Association and Royal Pharmaceutical Society.

Brotchie, Jane and Wann, Mai (1993) *Training for lay participation in health: Token voices or champions of the people?* London: The Patients Association.

Brown, Lesley (ed) (1993) *The new shorter Oxford dictionary on historical principles*, Oxford: Clarendon Press.

Brown, Phil (2000) 'Naming and framing: The social construction of diagnosis and illness', in Phil Brown (ed) *Perspectives in medical sociology* (3rd edn), Long Grove, IL: Waveland Press, Inc., pp 74–103.

Brown, Phil and Zavestoski, Stephen (2004) 'Social movements in health: An introduction', *Sociology of Health & Illness*, vol 26, no 6, pp 679–94.

Brown, Phil, Zavestoski, Stephen, McCormick, Sabrina, Mayer, Brian, Morello-Frosch, Rachel and Gasior Altman, Rebecca (2004) 'Embodied health movements: new approaches to social movements in health', *Sociology of Health & Illness*, vol 26, no 1, pp 50–80.

Brown, Rhoda F., Butow, Phyllis N., Sharrock, Merin Anne, Henman, Michael, Boyle, Fran, Goldstein, David and Tattersall, Martin H.N. (2004) 'Education and role modelling for clinical decisions with female cancer patients', *Health Expectations*, vol 7, no 4, pp 303–16.

Callery, Peter and Luker, Karen (1996) 'The use of qualitative methods in the study of parents' experiences of care on a children's ward', *Journal of Advanced Nursing*, vol 23, pp 338–45.

Calnan, Michael W. and Williams, Simon (1990) *Consumer satisfaction with health care, First stage 1989–1990*, Canterbury, Kent: Centre for Health Service Studies, University of Kent.

Campaign Against Hysterectomy and Unnecessary Operations on Women (1997) *Proposal for a woman's medical protection Act*, Woking, Surrey: Campaign Against Hysterectomy and Unnecessary Operations on Women.

Camus, Albert (1961) *Resistance, rebellion and death*, New York: Alfred A. Knopf.

Cang, Stephen (1978) 'Community health councils: Intentions, problems and possibilities', in E. Jaques (ed) *Health services, their nature and organisation and the role of patients, doctors and nurses and the complementary professions*, London: Heinemann, pp 267–78.

Carling, Margaret, Goodare, Heather, Ironside, Audrey, Millington, Jan and Rogers, Christina (2008) Letter, *The Lancet*, vol 372, p 204.

Chanter, Tina (2006) *Gender: Key concepts in philosophy*, London: Continuum International Publishing Group.

Chapman, G. (1999) 'Pre-operative autologous transfusion – the NBS experience', *Bulletin of the Royal College of Pathologists*, vol 105, p xiv.

Chatfield, C. and Collins, A.J. (1980) *Introduction to multivariate analysis*, London: Chapman and Hall.

Charles, Rachel (1996) 'Immune response', in Heather Goodare (ed) *Fighting spirit: The stories of women in the Bristol breast cancer survey*, London: Scarlet Press, pp 26–40.

Chochinov, H. (2007) 'Dignity and the essence of medicine: the A, B, C, and D of dignity conserving care', *British Medical Journal*, vol 335, pp 184–7.

Choonara, Imti (2004) 'Direct reporting of suspected adverse drug reactions by patients', *Journal of the Royal Society of Medicine*, vol 97, July, p 316.

Cohen, Gerda L. (1964) *What's wrong with hospitals?* Harmondsworth: Penguin Books Ltd.

Coldicott, Yvette, Pope, Catherine and Roberts, Clive (2003) 'The ethics of intimate examinations – teaching tomorrow's doctors', *BMJ*, vol 326, pp 97–101.

Conan Doyle, Arthur (1928) *Sherlock Holmes, The complete short stories*. London: John Murray, pp 305–33.

Conrad, Peter (2000) 'Medicalization and social control', in Phil Brown (ed) *Perspectives in medical sociology* (3rd edn), Long Grove, IL: Waveland Press, Inc., pp 104–29.

Coombes, Rebecca (2008) 'Healthcare Commission will publicise NHS trusts' levels of infection control', *BMJ*, vol 336, pp 526–7.

Coulter, Angela (2005) 'What do patients and the public want from primary care?', *BMJ*, vol 331, pp 1199–200.

Coulter, Angela, Entwistle, Vikki and Gilbert, David (1999) 'Sharing decisions with patients: Is the information good enough?' *BMJ*, vol 318, pp 318–22.

Coulter, Angela, Parsons, Suzanne and Askham, Janet (2008) *Where are the patients in decision-making about their own care?* Copenhagen: World Health Organisation.

Council for Science and Society (1980) *Childbirth today*, London: CSS.

Coyle, Joanne (1999) 'Understanding dissatisfied users: Developing a framework for comprehending criticisms of health care work', *Journal of Advanced Nursing*, vol 30, no 3, pp 723–31.

Crampsey, David P. (2009) '"I want to see the consultant"', *BMJ*, vol 338, p 955.

Crean, P[eter] M., Stokes M[onica] A., Williamson C[harlotte] and Hatch D[avid] J. (2003) 'Quality in paediatric anaesthesia: A pilot study of interdepartmental peer review', *Anaesthesia*, vol 58, pp 543–8.

Cropper, Gordon (2008) 'Book review', *The Bulletin of the Royal College of Pathologists*, vol 144, p 310.

Cross, Amanda [pseudonym of Carolyn Heilbrun] (1995) *An imperfect spy*, London: Virago.

Crossley, Michele L. and Crossley, Nick (2001) '"Patient" voices, social movements and the habitus; How psychiatric survivors "speak out"', *Social Science & Medicine*, vol 52, pp 1477–89.

Crow, Julie (2002) 'Royal College of Pathologists' advice relating to the ownership, storage and release of pathology results', *Bulletin of The Royal College of Pathologists*, vol 117, pp 33–4.

Dalrymple, Jane and Burke, Beverley (2006) *Anti-oppressive practice: Social care and the law*, Maidenhead: Open University Press.

Davies, Celia (2001) *Lay involvement in professional regulation: A study of public appointment-holders in the health field*, Milton Keynes: The School of Health and Social Welfare, The Open University, Open University Press.

Davies, E[lizabeth] and Cleary, P[aul] D. (2005) 'Hearing the patient's voice? Factors affecting the use of patient survey data in quality improvement', *Quality and Safety in Health Care*, vol 14, pp 428–32.

Davies, Myfanwy and Elwyn, Gwyn (2006) 'Referral management centres: Promising innovations or Trojan horses?', *BMJ*, vol 332, pp 844–6.

Davies, Tor (1997) 'Loveday demands colleges shape up', *Hospital Doctor*, 16 October, p 3.

Dearlove, John (1973) *The politics of policy in local government: The making and maintenance of public policy in the Royal Borough of Kensington and Chelsea*, London: Cambridge University Press.

Delamonthe, Tony (2008) 'A centrally funded health service, free at the point of delivery', *BMJ*, vol 336, pp 1410–12.

Dennis, Nancy (1988) 'A model of joint working', *Journal of the Royal College of General Practitioners*, November, p 491.

Department of Health (2000) *The NHS plan*, London: Department of Health.

Department of Health (2001) *Building a safer NHS for patients, Implementing an organisation with a memory*, London: Department of Health.

Department of Health (2003) *The new GMS contract*, London: Stationery Office.

DHSS (Department of Health and Social Security) (1969) *Report of the committee of inquiry into allegations of ill-treatment of patients and other irregularities at the Ely Hospital, Cardiff*, London: HMSO.

DHSS (1971) *Report of the Farleigh Hospital committee of inquiry*, London: HMSO.

DHSS (1972) *Report of the committee of inquiry into Whittingham Hospital*, London: HMSO.

DHSS (1974**a**) *Report of the committee of inquiry into South Ockendon Hospital*, London: HMSO.

DHSS (1974b) *Community health councils*, HRC (74)4.

DHSS (1978) *Report of the committee of inquiry into Normansfield Hospital*, London: HMSO.

DHSS and Welsh Office (1976) *The organisation of the in-patient's day*, London: Stationery Office.

Dixon-Woods, Mary (2001) 'Writing wrongs? An analysis of published discourses about the use of patient information leaflets', *Social Science & Medicine*, vol 52, pp1417–32.

Domizio, Paola (2008) 'I want to see my colon!' *Bulletin of the Royal College of Pathologists*, vol 142, p 123.

Doyal, Len and Wisher, Daniel (1993) 'Withholding cardiopulmonary resuscitation: Proposals for formal guidelines', *BMJ*, vol 306, pp 1593–6.

Durward, Lyn and Evans, Ruth (1990) 'Pressure groups and maternity care', in Jo Garcia, Robert Kilpatrick and Martin Richards (eds) *The politics of maternity care: Services for childbearing women in twentieth-century Britain*, Oxford: Clarendon Press, pp 256–73.

EACH (European Association for Children in Hospital) (2002) *The EACH charter & annotations*, London: EACH, www.each-for-sick-children.org.

Edwards, Adrian and Elwyn, Glyn (2006) 'Inside the black box of shared decision-making: Distinguishing between the process of involvement and who makes the decision', *Health Expectations*, vol 9, no 4, pp 307–20.

Edwards, Carol, Staniszweska, Sophie and Crichton, Nicola (2004) 'Investigation of the ways in which patients' reports of their satisfaction with healthcare are constructed', *Sociology of Health & Illness*, vol 26, no 2, pp 159–83.

Edwards, Nadine (2003) 'The choice is yours – or is it?' *AIMS Journal*, vol 15, no 3, pp 9–12.

Edwards, Nadine Pilley (2005) *Birthing autonomy: Women's experiences of planning home births*, Abingdon: Routledge.

Elledge, Richard M. and Osborne, C. Kent (1997) 'Oestrogen receptors and breast cancer', *BMJ*, vol 314, pp 1843–4.

Elliot-Smith, Adrian (2009) 'A final g'day to English general practice', *British Journal of General Practice*, vol 59, no 565, pp 618–20.

Elton, Charles (1942) 'Preface', *Voles, mice and lemmings*, Oxford: Clarendon Press.

Elwyn, Glyn (2006) 'Idealistic, impractical, impossible? Shared decision-making in the real world', *British Journal of General Practice*, vol 56, no 526, pp 403–4.

Elwyn, Glyn, Edwards, Adrian, Kinnersley, Paul and Grol, Richard (2000) 'Shared decision making and the concept of equipoise: The competences of involving patients in healthcare choices', *British Journal of General Practice*, vol 50, no 460, pp 892–7.

Enkin, Murray, Keirse, Marc J.N.C. and Chalmers, Iain (1989) *A guide to effective care in pregnancy and childbirth*, Oxford: Oxford University Press.

Entwistle, Vikki A. (2006) 'Considerations of "fit" and patient involvement in decision-making', *Health Expectations*, vol 9, no 2, pp 95–7.

Epstein, Steven (1996) *Impure science, AIDS, activism, and the politics of knowledge*, Berkeley, CA: University of California Press.

Fallberg, Lars H. and Calltorp, Johan (1999) 'Medical accidents and mishaps: the Swedish situation', in Marilynn M. Rosenthal, Linda Mulcahy and Sally Lloyd-Bostock (eds) *Medical mishaps: Pieces of the puzzle*, Buckingham: Open University Press, pp 84–94.

Farrell, Christine and Levitt, Ruth (1980) *Consumers, community health councils and the NHS*, London: King's Fund Centre.

Felski, Rita (2003) *Literature after feminism*, Chicago, IL: University of Chicago Press.

Firth, John (2007) 'Should you tell patients about beneficial treatments that they cannot have? No', *BMJ*, vol 334, p 827.

Fletcher, Colin (2002) 'Supervising activists for research degrees: responsibilities, rights and freedoms', *Active Learning for Higher Education*, vol 3, no 1, pp 88–103.

Flynn, Gordon (2006) 'Oh no, not again?' *BMJcareers*, 21 January, p 27.

Fox, Nicholas J. (1992) *The social meaning of surgery*, Milton Keynes: Open University Press.

Frampton, Susan, Guastello, Sara, Brady, Carrie, Hale, Maria, Horowitz, Sheryl, Bennett Smith, Susan and Stone, Susan (2008) *Patient-centered care improvement guide*, Derby, CT: Planetree, Inc.

Franklin, John Hope (1947) *From slavery to freedom, A history of negro Americans*, New York: Alfred A. Knopf.

Freedman, Jane (2001) *Feminism*, Buckingham: Open University Press.

Freidson, Eliot (1970a) *Professional dominance: The social structure of medical care*, New York: Aldine Publishing Company.

Freidson, Eliot (1970b) *Profession of medicine: A study of the sociology of applied knowledge*, New York: Dodd, Mead & Company.

Freidson, Eliot (2001) *Professionalism: The third logic.* Oxford: Polity Press and Blackwell Publishers Ltd.

Fried, Charles (1974) *Medical experimentation: Personal integrity and social policy*, New York: American Elsevier.

Fuchs Epstein, Cynthia (1988) *Deceptive distinctions, Sex, gender, and the social order*, New Haven and London: Yale University Press and New York: Russell Sage Foundation.

Furness, Peter N. (2003) 'Ethical aspects of histopathology', in D. Lowe and J. Underwood (eds) *Recent Advances in Histopathology*, vol 20, London: The Royal Society of Medicine Press, Limited, pp 115–28.

Furness, Peter (2007) 'Introducing new laboratory tests: the need for a new national strategy', *Bulletin of the Royal College of Pathologists*, vol 137, pp 34–5.

Gabe, Jonathan, Bury, Mike and Elston, Mary Ann (2004) *Key concepts in medical sociology*, London: Sage Publications Ltd.

Gawande, Atul (2004) 'On washing hands', *New England Journal of Medicine*, vol 350, no 13, pp 1283–6.

General Medical Council (1998) *Seeking patients' consent: The ethical considerations*, London: General Medical Council.

Gerrard, Mike (2006) *A stifled voice: Community health councils in England 1974–2003*, Brighton: Pen Press Publishers Ltd.

Gerteis, Margaret, Edgman-Levitan, Susan, Daley, Jennifer and Delbanco, Thomas (eds) (1993) *Through the patient's eyes: Understanding and promoting patient-centered care*, San Francisco, CA: Jossey-Bass Inc.

Gilbert, Hilary (1995) *Redressing the balance: A brief survey of literature on patient empowerment*, London: King's Fund Centre.

Gilligan, Carol (1982) *In a different voice: Psychological theory and women's development*, Cambridge, MA: Harvard University Press.

Goffman, Erving (1968) *Asylums: Essays on the social situation of mental patients and other inmates*, Harmondsworth: Penguin (first published in 1961 by Anchor Books, Doubleday & Co.).

Goodare, Heather (1996a) 'Introduction', in Heather Goodare (ed) *Fighting spirit: The stories of women in the Bristol breast cancer survey*, London: Scarlet Press, pp 1–10.

Goodare, Heather (1996b) 'The search for meaning', in Heather Goodare (ed) *Fighting spirit: The stories of women in the Bristol breast cancer survey*, London: Scarlet Press, pp 113–30.

Goodare, Heather (1996c) 'Coda', in Heather Goodare (ed) *Fighting spirit: The stories of women in the Bristol breast cancer survey*, London: Scarlet Press, pp 130–3.

Goodare, Heather (2007) 'The media and cancer survival', *Journal of the Royal Society of Medicine*, vol 100, pp 483–4.

Goodrich, Joanna and Cornwell, Jocelyn (2008) *Seeing the person in the patient*, London: King's Fund.

Goodwin, Jeff, Jasper, James M. and Polletta, Francesca (2001) *Passionate politics: Emotions and social movements*, Chicago, IL: University of Chicago Press.

Goodwin, Jeff, Jasper, James M. and Polletta, Francesca (2001a) 'Why emotions matter', in Jeff Goodwin, James M. Jasper and Francesca Polletta (2001) *Passionate politics: Emotions and social movements*, Chicago, IL: University of Chicago Press, pp 1-24.

Gould, Deborah (2001) 'Rock the boat, don't rock the boat, baby: ambivalence and the emergence of militant AIDS activism', in Jeff Goodwin, James M. Jasper and Francesca Polletta (eds) *Passionate politics: Emotions and social movements*, Chicago, IL: University of Chicago Press, pp 135–57.

Gould, Jonathan (ed) (1968) *The prevention of damaging stress in children. Report of UK study group no 1 to The World Federation for Mental Health*, London: J. & A. Churchill Ltd.

Graham, Hilary and Oakley, Ann (1989) 'Competing ideologies of reproduction: medical and maternal perspectives on pregnancy', in Elizabeth Whitelegg, Madeleine Arnot and Else Bartels (eds) *The changing experience of women*, Oxford: Basil Blackwell, pp 309–26 (first published in 1982).

Gray, Muir J.A. (2002) *The resourceful patient*, Oxford: eRosetta Press.

Greco, Peter J. and Eisenberg, John M. (1993) 'Changing physicians' practices', *New England Journal of Medicine*, vol 329, no 17, pp 1271–3.

Greenhalgh, Trisha and Wessely, Simon (2004) '"Health for me": a sociocultural analysis of healthism in the middle classes', *British Medical Bulletin*, vol 69, pp 197–213.

Grime, Janet, Blenkinsopp, Alison, Raynor, David K., Pollock, Kristian and Knapp, Peter (2007) 'The role and value of written information for patients about individual medicines: a sytematic review', *Health Expectations*, vol 10, no 3, pp 286–98.

Groch, Sharon (2001) 'Free spaces: creating oppositional consciousness in the disability rights movement', in Jane Mansbridge and Aldon Morris (eds) *Oppositional consciousness, The subjective roots of social protest*, Chicago, IL: University of Chicago Press, pp 65–98.

Grol, Richard (1999) 'Foreword', in Adrian Edwards and Glyn Elwyn (eds) *Evidence-based patient choice, Inevitable or impossible?* Oxford: Oxford University Press, pp xvi–xvii.

Groves, Julian McAllister (2001) 'Animal rights and the politics of emotion: folk constructs of emotion in the Animal Rights Movement', in Jeff Goodwin, James M. Jasper and Francesca Polletta (eds) *Passionate politics: Emotions and social movements*, Chicago, IL: University of Chicago Press, pp 212–29.

Hales-Tooke, Ann (1973) *Children in hospital: The parents' view*, London: Priory Press.

Hallas, Jack (1976) *CHCs in action*, London: Nuffield Provincial Hospitals Trust.

Halton, William (1994) 'Some unconscious aspects of organizational life: contributions from psychoanalysis', in Anton Obholzer and Vega Zagier Roberts (eds) *The unconscious at work: Individual and organizational stress in the human services*, London: Routledge, pp 11–18.

Ham, Christopher (1981) *Policy-making in the National Health Service*, London: The Macmillan Press Ltd.

Hancock, Sheila (1996) 'Foreword', in Heather Goodare (ed) *Fighting spirit: The stories of women in the Bristol breast cancer survey*, London: Scarlet Press, pp viii–x.

Hanley, Bec and Staley, Kristina (2006) *Yesterday's women, The story of R.A.G.E.*, London: Macmillan Cancer Support.

Harlow, H.E. and Harlow, M.K. (1961) 'A study of animal affection', *Natural History*, vol 70, pp 48–55.

Harrison, Philip J. (2008) 'Please don't forget ethical responsibilities', *BMJ*, vol 336, p 1085.

Harrison, Stephen and McDonald, Ruth (2008) *The politics of healthcare in Britain*, London: SAGE Publications Inc.

Harrison, Stephen and Pollitt, Christopher (1994) *Controlling health professionals,: The future of work and organization in the NHS*, Buckingham: Open University Press.

Harrison, Stephen, Hunter, David J. and Pollitt, Christopher (1990) *The dynamics of British health policy*, London: Routledge.

Haug, Marie R. and Sussman, Marvin B. (1969) 'Professional autonomy and the revolt of the client', *Social Problems*, vol 17, pp 153–61.

Healthcare Commission (2005) *Survey of patients 2005, Stroke*, London: Healthcare Commission.

Healthcare Commission (2007) *Women's experiences of maternity care in the NHS in England*, London: Commission for Healthcare Audit and Inspection.

Healthcare Commission (2009) *Investigation into Mid Staffordshire NHS Foundation Trust*, London: Healthcare Commission.

Heilbrun, Carolyn G. (1964) *Towards a recognition of androgyny*, New York: Alfred A. Knopf.

Heilbrun, Carolyn G. (1989) *Writing a woman's life*, London: The Woman's Press (first published New York, W.W. Norton, 1988).

Heilbrun, Carolyn G. (1990) *Hamlet's mother and other women*, New York: Ballantyne Books.

Help the Aged (2008) *On our own terms: The challenge of assessing dignity in care*, London: Help the Aged.

Heneghan, Christopher P.H. (1999) 'Critical incidents – to tell or not to tell?', *Royal College of Anaesthetists Newsletter*, vol 46, pp 115–16.

Herxheimer, Andrew (2003) 'Relationships between the pharmaceutical industry and patients' organisations', *BMJ*, vol 326, pp 1208–10.

Herxheimer, Andrew (2005) 'Talking about harms and risks', *Health Expectations*, vol 8, no 4, pp 283–5.

Hess, David J. (2004) 'Medical modernisation, scientific research fields and the epistemic politics of health social movements', *Sociology of Health & Illness*, vol 26, no 6, pp 695–709.

Hindley, Carol and Thomson, Ann M. (2005) 'The rhetoric of informed choice: perspectives from midwives on intrapartum fetal heart rate monitoring', *Health Expectations*, vol 8, no 4, pp 306–14.

Hingorani, Melanie, Wong, Tina and Vafidis, Gilli (1999) 'Patients' and doctors' attitudes to the amount of information given after unintended injury during treatment: cross sectional, questionnaire study', *BMJ*, vol 318, p 640.

Hirst, Jenny (1997/98) 'Consumer involvement dream or reality?' *CERES Newsletter*, Winter 97/98, no 23, pp 4–7.

Hirst, Jenny (2002) 'At last – the high quality evidence!', *Insulin Dependent Diabetes Trust October 2002 Newsletter*, no 34, pp 1–2.

Hirst, Jenny (2003) '"Dead in bed" syndrome', *Insulin Dependent Diabetes Trust July 2003 Newsletter*, no 37, p 4.

Hirst, Jenny (2004) '2004 – IDDT's 10th anniversary, A time for celebration or sadness?' *Insulin Dependent Diabetes Trust January 2004 Newsletter*, no 39, p 1.

Hirst, Jenny (2005a) 'Not listening to what patients say – is it instinctive?', *Insulin Dependent Diabetes Trust April 2005 Newsletter*, no 44, pp 1–2.

Hirst, Jenny (2005b) 'Is IDDT the naughty child of diabetes organisations?', *Insulin Dependent Diabetes Trust July 2005 Newsletter*, no 45, pp 1–2.

Hock, Y.L., Balachander, C., Dicken, S., Bayley, C. and Ramaiah, S. (2005) 'Patients' perspective of pathology specimens, a prospective study', *Journal of Clinical Pathology*, vol 58, pp 891–3.

Hogg, Christine (1988) *Frontier medicine, New medical techniques and the consumer*, London: Greater London Association of Community Health Councils.

Hogg, Christine (1999) *Patients, power and politics, From patients to citizens*, London: SAGE Publications Ltd.

Hogg, Christine (2009) *Citizens, consumers and the NHS: Capturing voices,* Basingstoke: Palgrave Macmillan.

Hogg, Christine and Rodin, Jo (1989) *The NAWCH quality review: Setting standards for children in hospital,* London: NAWCH.

Hogg, Christine and Williamson, Charlotte (2001) 'Whose interests do lay people represent? Towards an understanding of the role of lay people as members of committees', *Health Expectations,* vol 4, no 1, pp 2–9.

Holland, Paul V. (1999) 'Viral infections and the blood supply', *New England Journal of Medicine,* vol 334, no 26, pp 1734–5.

Hooper, D. (2008) Letter, 'The PLG debates', *Bulletin of the Royal College of Anaesthetists,* vol 48, p 2472.

Howard, Martin R., Chapman, Catherine E., Dunston, Judith A,. Mitchell, Christine and Lloyd, Huw L. (1992) 'Regional transfusion centre for pre-operative autologous blood transfusion: the first two years', *BMJ,* vol 305, pp 1470–3.

IDDT (Insulin Dependent Diabetic Trust) (2006) 'Notice', in *British Journal of General Practice,* vol 56, no 529, p 626.

Inman, Bill (1999) *Don't tell the patient: Behind the drug safety net,* Los Angeles, CA: Highland Park Productions.

Irvine, Donald (2003) *The doctors' tale: Professionalism and public trust,* Abingdon: Radcliffe Medical Press Ltd.

James, P[hyllis] D. (2008) *The private patient,* London: Faber and Faber Limited.

Jensen, Uffe Juul and Mooney, Gavin (1990) 'Changing values: autonomy and paternalism in medicine and health care', in U.J. Jensen and G. Mooney (eds) *Changing values in medical and health care decision making,* Chichester: John Wiley & Sons, pp 1–15.

Johnson, Terence J. (1972) *Professions and power,* London: The Macmillan Press Ltd.

Jolley, M.G. (1988) 'Ethics of cancer management from the patient's perspective', *Journal of Medical Ethics,* vol 14, no 4, pp 188–90.

Jorm, Christine and Kam, Peter (2004) 'Does medical culture limit doctors' adoption of quality improvement? Lessons from Camelot', *Journal of Health Service Research Policy,* vol 9, no 4, pp 248–51.

Kemper, Theodore D. (2001) 'A structural approach to social movement emotions', in Jeff Goodwin, James M. Jasper and Francesca Polletta (eds) *Passionate politics: Emotions and social movements,* Chicago, IL: University of Chicago Press, pp 58–73.

Kestin, I. (2007) 'Letters to the Editor', *Bulletin of the Royal College of Anaesthetists,* vol 46, pp 2367–8.

Kieve, Millie (2004) 'She told me she had lost her personality', www.guardian.co.uk.healthstory.

Kieve, Millie (2006) 'APRIL charity 2006', www.april.org.uk.

King, Margaret (1997) 'Presentation to the UK National Breast Cancer Coalition's research committee on 30 January 1997 on radiotherapy and the START trial', in *[Report of] UKNBCC workshop held at Bristol Cancer Centre*, London: UK National Breast Coalition.

Klandermans, Bert (1997) *The social psychology of protest*, Oxford: Blackwell Publishers Ltd.

Klein, Rudolf (1993) 'Dimensions of rationing: who should do what?', *BMJ*, vol 307, pp 309–11.

Klein, Rudolf and Lewis, Janet (1976) *The politics of consumer representation, A study of Community Health Councils*, London: Centre for Studies in Social Policy.

Koch-Weser, Susan, Dejong, William and Rudd, Rime E. (2009) 'Medical word use in clinical encounters', *Health Expectations*, vol 12, no 4, pp 371–82.

Kravitz, Richard L. and Melnikow, Joy (2001) 'Engaging patients in medical decision making', *BMJ*, vol 323, pp 584–5.

Krebs, Susan (1997) *Carolyn G. Heilbrun, Feminist in a tenured position*, Charlottesville, VA: The University Press of Virginia.

Krumholz, Harlan M., Ross, Joseph S., Coutts, Gordon, Tiner, Richard, Angell, Marcia and Gottlieb, Scott (2009) 'Doctors, patients and the drug industry: partners, friends or foes?', *BMJ*, vol 338, pp 326–9.

Lack, J. Alastair (2003) 'Chairman's Introduction – Information for patients', in J. Alastair Lack, Anna-Maria Rollin, Gavin Thoms, Lucy White and Charlotte Williamson (eds) *Raising the standard: Information for patients*, London: Royal College of Anaesthetists and Association of Anaesthetists of Great Britain and Ireland, pp 5–6.

Lack, J. Alastair, Rollin, Anna-Maria, Thoms, Gavin, White, Lucy and Williamson, Charlotte (eds) (2003) *Raising the standard: Information for patients*, London: Royal College of Anaesthetists and Association of Anaesthetists of Great Britain and Ireland.

Lavelle-Jones, Christine, Byrne, Derek J., Rice, Peter and Cuschieri, Alfred (1993) 'Factors affecting quality of informed consent', *BMJ*, vol 306, pp 885–90.

Learmonth, Mark, Martin, Graham P. and Warwick, Philip (2009) 'Ordinary and effective: the Catch-22 in managing the public voice in health care?', *Health Expectations*, vol 12, no 1, pp 106–15.

Lee, John (2005) 'A medical perspective', *Bulletin of The Royal College of Pathologists*, vol 130, pp 59–60.

Levenson, Ros and Joule, Nikki (1999) *Improving people's lives, The agenda for people with long-term medical conditions*, London: The Long-term Medical Alliance.

Leydon, Geraldine M., Boulton, Mary, Moynihan, Clare, Jones, Alison, Mossman, Jean, Boudioni, Markella and McPherson, Klim (2000) 'Cancer patients' information needs and information seeking behaviour: in depth interview study', *BMJ*, vol 320, pp 909–13.

Lister, Sam (2004) 'GPs foil attempt to make letters available for patients' scrutiny', *The Times*, 29 April.

Little, Miles, Jordens, Christopher F.C., Paul, Kim, Sayers, Emma-Jane, Cruickshank, Jane Ann, Stegeman, Jantine and Montgomery, Kathleen (2002) 'Discourse in different voices: reconciling N=1 and N=many', *Social Science & Medicine*, vol 55, pp 1979–87.

Little, William, Fowler, H.W. and Coulson, J. (1936) *The shorter Oxford English dictionary on historical principles*, Oxford: Clarendon Press, second edition.

Lloyd-Bostock, Sally (1999) 'Calling doctors and hospitals to account: complaining and claiming as social processes', in Marilynn M. Rosenthal, Linda Mulcahy and Sally Lloyd-Bostock (eds) *Medical mishaps: Pieces of the puzzle*, Buckingham: Open University Press, pp 109–23.

Lomas, Jonathan (1993) 'Retailing research: increasing the role of evidence in clinical services for childbirth', *The Milbank Quarterly*, vol 71, no 3, pp 439–75.

Lown, Beth A., Hanson, Janice L. and Clark, William D. (2009) 'Mutual influence in shared decision making: a collaborative study of patients and physicians', *Health Expectations*, vol 12, no 2, pp 160–74.

Lukes, Steven (2005) *Power: A radical view* (2nd edn), Basingstoke: Palgrave Macmillan (1st edn, 1974).

McCaughrin, William Cass (1994) 'Perspective: riddles wrapped in enigma', *Journal of Health Care Quality*, vol 16, no 1, pp 30–7.

McColl, E[laine] (2005) 'I just want the protocol, doctor!' *Quality & Safety in Health Care*, vol 14, p 155.

McCullough, Laurence B. (1988) 'An ethical model for improving the patient–physician relationship', *Inquiry*, vol 25, Winter, pp 454–65.

Macintyre, Sally and Oldman, David (1977) 'Coping with migraine', in Alan Davis and Gordon Horobin (eds) *Medical encounters: The experience of illness and treatment*, London: Croom Helm, pp 55–71.

Mach, Ernst (1883) *The science of mechanics: A critical and historical account of its development* (5th edn), La Salle, IL: The Open Court Publishing Company.

Mansbridge, Jane (2001a) 'The making of oppositional consciousness', in Jane Mansbridge and Aldon Morris (eds) *Oppositional consciousness: The subjective roots of social protest*, Chicago, IL: University of Chicago Press, pp 1–19.

Mansbridge, Jane (2001b) 'Complicating oppositional consciousness', in Jane Mansbridge and Aldon Morris (eds) *Oppositional consciousness, The subjective roots of social protest*, Chicago, IL: University of Chicago Press, pp 238–64.

Marcus, Robert (2007) 'Should you tell patients about beneficial treatments that they cannot have? Yes', *BMJ*, vol 334, pp 826.

Marriott, F.H.C. (1974) *The interpretation of multiple observations*, London: Academic Press, Inc.

Marsh, B.T. (1987) 'Be a patient', *BMJ*, vol 295, pp 909–10.

Martin, Graham P. (2008) '"Ordinary people only": knowledge, representativeness, and the publics of public participation in healthcare', *Sociology of Health & Illness*, vol 30, no 1, pp 35–54.

Martin, Margaret and White, Lucy (2003) 'A review of other resources', in J. Alastair Lack, Anna-Maria Rollin, Gavin Thoms, Lucy White and Charlotte Williamson (eds) *Raising the standard: Information for patients*, London: Royal College of Anaesthetists and Association of Anaesthetists of Great Britain and Ireland, pp 136–42.

Mechanic, David (2004) 'In my chosen doctor I trust', *BMJ*, vol 329, pp 1418–19.

Medawar, Charles and Hardon, Anita (2004) *Medicines out of control? Antidepressants and the conspiracy of goodwill*, The Netherlands: Aksant Academic Publishers.

MHRA (Medicines and Healthcare products Regulatory Agency) (2004) *Annual report and accounts 2003*, London: The Stationery Office.

Menzies, Isabel E.P. (1959) 'The functioning of social systems as a defence against anxiety: a report on a study of the nursing service in a general hospital', *Human Relations*, vol 13, pp 95–121.

Menzies Lyth, Isabel (1988a) 'Reflections on my work, Isabel Menzies Lyth in conversation with Ann Scott and Robert M. Young', in Isabel Menzies Lyth *Containing anxiety in institutions, Selected essays*, vol 1, London: Free Association Books, pp 1–42.

Menzies Lyth, Isabel (1988b) 'Action research in a long-stay hospital', in Isabel Menzies Lyth *Containing anxiety in institutions, Selected essays*, vol 1, pp 130–52.

MIDIRS and the NHS Centre for Reviews and Dissemination (1996) *Informed choice leaflets: Using evidence to empower childbearing women*, Bristol: MIDIRS and NHS Centre for Reviews and Dissemination.

Miles, Rosalind (1988) *The women's history of the world*, London: Michael Joseph.

Milne, Rhairidh, Booth-Clibborn, Nina and Oliver, Sandy (2000), Letter 'Consumer health information needs to be rigorous, complete and relevant', *BMJ*, vol 321, p 240.

Ministry of Health (1959) *The welfare of children in hospital: The report of the committee (The Platt Report)*, London: HMSO.

Mol, Annemarie (2008) *The logic of care: Health and the problem of patient choice*, London: Routledge.

Moore, Jane, Ziebland, Sue, Stephen (2002) '"People sometimes react funny if they're not told enough": women's views about the risks of diagnostic laparoscopy', *Health Expectations*, vol 5, no 4, pp 302–9.

Moore, Peter and Roland, Martin (2008) 'Should GPs be paid to cut hospital referrals?', *The Times*, 31 October, p 65.

Munro, A.J. (2007) 'Hidden danger, obvious opportunity: error and risk in the management of cancer', *British Journal of Radiology*, vol 80, pp 955–66.

National Association for the Welfare of Children in Hospital (1990) *Update 1970–1990*, London: NAWCH

National Blood Service (2002) *Receiving a blood transfusion*, London: NBS.

National Consumer Council (1996) *Putting it right for consumers*, London: National Consumer Council.

National Health and Medical Research Council (2000) *How to prepare and present evidence-based information for consumers of health services: A literature review (1999)*, Canberra: Commonwealth of Australia.

NCEPOD (National Confidential Enquiry into Patient Outcome and Death) (2008) *For better, for worse? A review of the care of patients who died within 30 days of receiving systemic anti-cancer therapy*, London: NCEPOD.

Nehamas, N. (1957) *Nietzsche: Life as literature*, Cambridge, MA: Harvard University Press.

New, Bill and Le Grand, Julian (1996) *Rationing in the NHS, Principles and pragmatism*, London: King's Fund Publishing.

Newton, Kenneth (1976) *Second city politics: Democratic processes and decision-making in Birmingham*, Oxford: Clarendon Press.

Nicol, Nicholas (1999) 'The right to redress: complaints and principles of grievance procedures', in Marilynn M. Rosenthal, Linda Mulcahy and Sally Lloyd-Bostock (eds) *Medical mishaps: Pieces of the puzzle*, Buckingham: Open University Press, pp 239–45.

North, Nancy (1995) 'Alford revisited: the professional monopolisers, corporate rationalisers, community and markets', *Policy and Politics*, vol 23, no 2, pp 115–25.

North, Nancy and Peckham, Stephen (2001) 'Analysing structural interests in primary care groups', *Social Policy & Administration*, vol 35, no 4, pp 426–40.

Obama, Barack (2009) 'The inauguration speech, President Obama, 20 January 2009', *The Times Supplement, Obama, The inauguration*, pp 10–11.

Offe, Claus (1984) *Contradictions of the welfare state*, edited by John Keane, London: Hutchinson.

Oliver, Sandy, Milne, Rhairidh, Bradbury, Jane, Buchanan, Phyllis, Kerridge, Lynn, Walley, Tom and Gabbay, John (2001) 'Involving consumers in the needs-led research programme: a pilot project', *Health Expectations*, vol 4, no 1, pp 18–28.

Olszewski, Deborah and Jones, Lyn (1998) *Putting people in the picture, Information for patients and the public about illness and treatment*, Edinburgh: Scottish Association of Health Councils and Scottish Health Feedback.

PACE Angina Project (nd but prior to 2003) *Looking after your angina*, South Tyneside: PACE.

Parroy, Susan, Thoms, Gavin and Williamson, Charlotte (2003) 'The practicalities of developing patient information', in J. Alastair Lack, Anna-Maria Rollin, Gavin Thoms, Lucy White and Charlotte Williamson (eds) *Raising the standard: Information for patients*, London: Royal College of Anaesthetists and Association of Anaesthetists of Great Britain and Ireland, pp 15–23.

Parsons, Talcott (1951) *The social system*, London: Routledge and Kegan Paul.

Pellegrino, Edmund D. and Thomasma, David C. (1981) *A philosophical basis of medical practice: Towards a philosophy and ethic of the healing professions*, New York: Oxford University Press.

Philips, Adam (1988) *Winnicott*, London: Fontana Press.

Picker Institute (2007) *Policy research primer*, Oxford: Picker Institute Europe.

Pierson, Paul (2004) *Politics in time: History, institutions, and social analysis*, Princeton, NJ: Princeton University Press.

Pitkin, Hanna F. (1967) *The concept of representation*, Berkeley, CA: University of California Press.

Polletta, Francesca and Amenta, Edwin (2001) 'Second that emotion?: Lessons from once-novel concepts in social movement research', in Jeff Goodwin, James M. Jasper and Francesca Polletta (eds) *Passionate politics: Emotions and social movements*, Chicago, IL: University of Chicago Press, pp 303–16.

Potter, Jenny (1988) 'Consumerism and the public sector: how well does the coat fit?', *Public Administration*, vol 66, Summer, pp 149–64.

Poulson, Jane (1998) 'Bitter pills to swallow', *New England Journal of Medicine*, vol 338, no 25, pp 1844–6.

Pyper, Cecilia, Amery, Justin, Watson, Marion and Crook, Claire (2004) 'Patients' experiences when accessing their on-line electronic patient records in primary care', *British Journal of General Practice*, vol 54, no 498, pp 38–43.

Quill, Timothy E. and Brody, Howard (1996) 'Physician recommendations and patient autonomy: finding a balance between physician power and patient choice', *Annals of Internal Medicine*, vol 125, no 9, pp 763–9.

Radcliffe, Mark (2004) 'Choice cuts, dissecting the policies', *BMA News*, 28 August, pp 6–7.

RAGE (Radiotherapy Action Group Exposure) (1997) *RAGE's response to 'The report of the independent review commissioned by the Royal College of Radiologists into brachial plexus neuropathy following radiotherapy for breast carcinoma'*, Bromley: RAGE.

RAGE (2007) 'Dear members and friends', *Radiotherapy Action Group Exposure Autumn Newsletter*, p 1.

Rees Jones, Ian, Berney, Lee, Kelly, Moira, Doyal, Len, Griffiths, Chris, Curtis, Sarah, Feder, Gene, Hillier, Sheila and Rowlands, Gillian (2004) 'Is patient involvement possible when decisions involve scarce resources? A qualitative study of decision-making in primary care', *Social Science & Medicine*, vol 59, pp 93–102.

Reeves, R[achel] and Seccombe, I[an] (2008) 'Do patient surveys work? The influence of a national survey programme on local quality-improvement initiatives', *Quality and Safety in Health Care*, vol 17, pp 437–41.

Resnik, Susan (1999) *Blood saga: Hemophilia, AIDS and the survival of a community*, Berkeley, CA: University of California Press.

Richards, Nick and Coulter, Angela (2007) *Is the NHS becoming more patient-centred? Trends from the national surveys of NHS patients in England 2002–07*, Oxford: Picker Institute Europe.

Richardson, Ruth (2001) 'Statement of Dr R. Richardson', in *Chief Medical Officer's Summit, Evidence documentation, 11th January 2001*, London: Health Services Directorate, no page numbers.

Rier, David A. (2000) 'The missing voice of the critically ill: a medical sociologist's first-person account', *Sociology of Health & Illness*, vol 22, no 1, pp 68–93.

Robb, Barbara (1967) 'Preface', in Barbara Robb (ed, *Sans everything: A case to answer*, London: Thomas Nelson and Sons Ltd, pp xiii–xvi.

Robertson, James (1953) *A two-year-old goes to hospital*, Tavistock Clinic [London] and New York: New York University Film Library.

Robertson, James (1958) *Young children in hospital*, London: Tavistock Publications.

Robertson, James (1961), in *The Observer*, 13, 22, 29 January.

Robertson, James (1989) 'Involving the community', in James Robertson and Joyce Robertson (eds), *Separation and the very young*, London: Free Association Books, pp 68–72.

Robinson, Jean (1985) 'Are we teaching students that patients don't matter?', *Journal of Medical Ethics*, vol 11, no 1, pp 15–21.

Robinson, Jean (1988) *A patient voice at the GMC: A lay member's view of the General Medical Council*, London: Health Rights Ltd.

Robinson, Jean (1993) 'Health service users and research', *CERES News*, vol 12, Autumn, pp 5–6.

Robinson, Jean (1996a) 'Dangerous therapy', *THS* [*Times Health Supplement*], October, pp 8–9.

Robinson, Jean (1996b) 'It's only a questionnaire ... ethics in social science research', *British Journal of Midwifery*, vol 4, no 1, pp 41–4.

Robinson, Jean (1999) 'The price of deceit: the reflections of an advocate', in Marilynn M. Rosenthal, Linda Mulcahy and Sally Lloyd-Bostock (eds) *Medical mishaps: Pieces of the puzzle*, Buckingham: Open University Press, pp 247–56.

Robinson, Jean (2004/5) 'Shooting the messenger', *AIMS Journal*, vol 16, no 4 p 15.

Rodger, Alan (1998) 'Fears over radiotherapy fractionation regimes in breast cancer', *BMJ*, vol 317, pp 155–6.

Rogers, Anne and Pilgrim, David (1991) '"Pulling down churches"; accounting for the British Mental Health Users' Movement', *Sociology of Health & Illness*, vol 13, no 2, pp 129–48.

Rogers, Wendy A. (2007) 'The tangled web of medical and commercial interests', *Health Expectations*, vol 10, no 1, pp 1–3.

Rollin, Anna-Maria (2003) 'The development of specialist booklets', in J. Alastair Lack, Anna-Maria Rollin, Gavin Thoms, Lucy White and Charlotte Williamson (eds) *Raising the standard: Information for patients*, London: Royal College of Anaesthetists and Association of Anaesthetists of Great Britain and Ireland, pp 24–9.

Rose, David (2008) 'Pointless NHS system becomes less rigid', *The Times*, 22 September, p 13.

Rosenthal, Marilynn M., Mulcahy, Linda and Lloyd-Bostock, Sally (eds) (1999) *Medical mishaps: Pieces of the puzzle*, Buckingham: Open University Press.

Ross, N[icki] (2009) 'The other side of the fence', *Bulletin of the Royal College of Anaesthetists*, vol 53, pp 20–2.

Rowbotham, Sheila (2004) 'Introduction', in Helene Curtis and Mimi Sanderson (eds) *The unsung sixties: Memoirs of social innovation*, London: Whiting & Birch Ltd, pp ix–xii.

Royal College of Anaesthetists and Association of Anaesthetists of Great Britain and Ireland (2002) *Anaesthesia explained: Information for patients, relatives and friends*, London: RCA and AAGBI.

Royal College of General Practitioners (1997a) *How to work with your doctor: Report of a project of the Royal College of General Practitioners' Patients Liaison Group*, Exeter: RCGP.

Royal College of General Practitioners (1997b) *Removal of patients from GPs' lists: Guidance for college members*, London: RCGP.

Royal College of Obstetricians and Gynaecologists (2001) *The national sentinel audit*, London: RCOG.

Royal Liverpool Children's Inquiry (2001) *The Royal Liverpool Children's inquiry report*, London: Stationery Office.

Ryder, Sandra (2007/8) 'Birth in Poole', *AIMS Journal*, vol 19, no 4, pp 21–2.

Salter, Brian (1999) 'Change in the governance of medicine: the politics of self-regulation', *Policy & Politics*, vol 27, no 2, pp 143–58.

Salter, Brian (2003) 'Patients and doctors: reformulating the UK health policy community?', *Social Science & Medicine*, vol 57, pp 927–36.

Salter, Brian (2004) *The new politics of medicine*, Basingstoke: Palgrave Macmillan.

Savage, Wendy (1986) *A savage enquiry: Who controls childbirth?* London, Virago Press.

Savage, Wendy (1990) 'How obstetrics might change: Wendy Savage talks to Robert Kilpatrick', in Jo Garcia, Robert Kilpatrick and Martin Richards (eds) *The politics of maternity care: Services for childbearing women in twentieth-century Britain*, Oxford: Clarendon Press, pp 325–40.

Schneider, Carl E. (1998) *The practice of autonomy: Patients, doctors, and medical decisions*, New York: Oxford University Press.

Schutz, Alfred (1964) 'The well-informed citizen, an essay on the social distribution of knowledge', in A. Brodersen (ed) *Alfred Schutz, Collected Papers II*, The Hague: Martinus Nijhoff, pp 120–34.

Sedgwick, Peter (1982) *Psycho politics*, London: Pluto Press.

Sen, Amartya (2009) *The idea of justice*, London: Allen Lane.

Seymour, Ann (2004) 'Obstetric anaesthesia', *Bulletin of the Royal College of Anaesthetists*, vol 25, p 1239.

Sharp, Imogen (1998) 'Gender issues in the prevention and treatment of coronary heart disease', in Lesley Doyle (ed) *Women and health services*, Buckingham: Open University Press, pp 100–12.

Sharrock, Wes and Watson, Rod (1995) 'The incarnation of social structure', in Patrick Joyce (ed) *Class*, Oxford: Oxford University Press, pp 108–13.

Shaw, Joanne (2009) 'A reformation for our times', *BMJ*, vol 338, p 719.

Sherwin, Susan (1992) *No longer patient: Feminist ethics and health care*, Philadelphia, PA: Temple University Press.

Sikora, Karol (1994) 'Enraged about radiotherapy', *BMJ*, vol 308, pp 188–9.

Sinclair, Frauke (2008) 'In need of TLC? A doctor–patient relationship fit for the future?', www.scottishcouncilfoundation.org, accessed 14 April 2008.

Sisk, Jane E. (1993) 'Improving the use of research-based evidence in policy-making: Effective Care in Pregnancy and Childbirth in the United States', *Milbank Quarterly*, vol 71, no 3, pp 477–96.

Skene, Loane and Smallwood, Richard (2002) 'Informed consent: lessons from Australia', *BMJ*, vol 324, pp 29–41.

Smith, Andrew F. (2003) Editorial, 'Patient information, risk and choice', *Anaesthesia*, vol 58, no 5, pp 409–11.'

Smith, Andrew and Adams, Tony (2003) 'Risk communication and anaesthesia', in J. Alastair Lack, Anna-Maria Rollin, Gavin Thoms, Lucy White and Charlotte Williamson (eds) *Raising the standard: Information for patients*, London: Royal College of Anaesthetists and Association of Anaesthetists of Great Britain and Ireland, pp 77–86.

Sokol, Daniel K. (2007) 'What would you do, doctor?', *BMJ*, vol 334, p 853.

Spriggs, Merle (1998) 'Autonomy in the face of a devastating diagnosis', *Journal of Medical Ethics*, vol 24, no 2, pp 123-6.

Spry, N.A., Lamb, D.S. and Dady, P.J. (1993) Letter, 'Resource restraints: what do we tell our patients?', *BMJ*, vol 307, p 559.

Stapleton, Helen, Kirkham, Mavis and Thomas, Gwenan (2002) 'Qualitative study of evidence based leaflets in maternity care', *BMJ*, vol 324, pp 639–43.

[The] START Trialists' Group (2008) 'The UK standardisation of breast radiotherapy (START) trial A of radiotherapy hypofractionation for treatment of early breast cancer: a randomised trial', *Lancet Oncology*, vol 9, pp 331–41.

Steering Committee for the Review of Access to Yellow Card Data (2004) *Report of an independent review of access to the Yellow Card Scheme*, London: The Stationery Office.

Steinbrook, Robert (2006) 'Imposing personal responsibility for health', *New England Journal of Medicine*, vol 355, no 8, pp 753–6.

Stevenson, R[obert] L[ouis] (1887) *Underwoods*, Chatto and Windus.

Stewart, Moira, Brown, Judith Belle, Weston, W. Wayne, McWhinney, Ian R., McWilliam, Carol L. and Freeman, Thomas R. (2003) *Patient-centered medicine: Transforming the clinical method*, Abingdon: Radcliffe Medical Press (1st edn 1995).

Stimpson, J. (2007) 'Letters to the Editor', *Bulletin of the Royal College of Anaesthetists*, vol 46, pp 2368–9.

Stimson, Gerry and Webb, Barbara (1975) *Going to see the doctor*, London: Routledge & Kegan Paul.

Strauss, Anselm L. and Glaser, Barney G. (1997) *Anguish: A case history of a dying trajectory*, London: Martin Robertson & Company, Ltd. (published in US in 1970).

Stubbs, Sonja K. (2001) 'Autologous donation – a patient's story', *Blood Matters*, vol 8, pp 4–5.

Suttie, Ian, D. (1960) *The origins of love and hate*, Harmondsworth: Penguin Books Ltd.

Tallis, Raymond (2004) *Hippocratic oaths: Medicine and its discontents*, London: Atlantic Books.

Tanne, Janice Hopkins (2009) 'Older US women are less likely than men to get kidney transplants', *BMJ*, vol 338, p 128.

Tattersall, Martin and Ellis, Peter (1998) 'Communication is a vital part of care', *BMJ*, vol 316, pp 1891–2.

Taylor, Pat and Lupton, Carol (1995) *Consumer involvement in health care commissioning*, Portsmouth: Social Sciences Research and Information Unit, University of Portsmouth.

Tew, Marjorie (1990) *Safer childbirth: A critical history of maternity care*. London: Chapman & Hall.

Thomas, Carol (2007) *Sociologies of disability and illness: Contested ideas in disability studies and medical sociology*, Basingstoke: Palgrave Macmillan.

Thomas, Pat (2002) 'The midwife you have called knows you are waiting', *AIMS Journal*, vol 14, no 3, pp 6–8.

Thornton, Hazel (2002) Letter, 'Debate is essential, not futile', *BMJ*, vol 324, p 110.

Thornton, Hazel, Edwards, Adrian and Elwyn, Glyn (2003) 'Evolving the multiple roles of "patients" in health-care research: reflections after involvement in a trial of shared decision-making', *Health Expectations*, vol 6, no 3, pp 189–97.

Toch, Hans (1965) *The social psychology of social movements*, Indianapolis, IN: The Bobbs-Merrill Company Inc.

Tong, Rosemarie (1997) *Feminist approaches to bioethics: Theoretical reflections and practical applications*, Boulder, CO: Westview Press.

Touraine, Alain (1995) 'Sociology and the study of society', in Patrick Joyce (ed) *Class*, Oxford: Oxford University Press, pp 83–9.

Trollope, Anthony (1995) *Barchester Towers*, London: The Folio Society (first published in 1857).

Tuckett, David, Boulton, Mary, Olson, Coral and Williams, Anthony (1985) *Meetings between experts: An approach to sharing ideas in medical consultations*, London: Tavistock Publications.

Tudor Hart, Julian (1998) 'Expectations of health care: promoted, managed or shared?' *Health Expectations*, vol 1, no 1, pp 3–13.

Tylko, Katherine and Blennerhassett, Mitzi (2006) 'How the NHS could better protect the safety of radiotherapy patients', *Health Care Risk Report*, September, pp 18–19.

Uddin, Shahana (2006) 'Patient safety comes second?', *BMJcareers*, 21 January, p 28.

Underwood, James (2003) 'From the President', *Bulletin of the Royal College of Pathologists*, vol 124, pp 3–4.

Underwood, James (2009) 'Human tissue legislation in the United Kingdom: the need and prospects for amendment', *Bulletin of the Royal College of Pathologists*, vol 147, pp 198–203.

Vaitheeswaran, Vijay (2009) 'Medicine goes digital, a special report on health care and technology', *The Economist*, vol 391, April 18, pp 3–16 of special report, inserted after p 54.

Vaizey, John (1959) *Scenes from institutional life*, London: Faber and Faber.

Wagner, Marsden (1994) *Pursuing the birthing machine, The search for appropriate birth technology*, Camperdown, NSW, Australia: ACE Graphics.

Waite, Lori G. (2001) 'Divided consciousness: the impact of black elite consciousness on the 1996 Chicago Freedom Movement', in Jane Mansbridge and Aldon Morris (eds) *Oppositional consciousness: The subjective roots of social protest*, Chicago, IL: University of Chicago Press, pp 170–203.

Waitzkin, Howard (2000) *The second sickness, Contradictions of capitalist health care* (2nd edn), Oxford: London: Rowman & Littlefield Publishers, Inc.

Wallston, Kenneth A. and Wallston, Barbara Strudler (1982) 'Who is responsible for your health? The construct of health locus of control', in Glennis S. Sanders and Jerry Sules (eds) *Social psychology of health and illness*, Hillsdale, NJ: Lawrence Erlbaum Associates, Publishers, pp 65–95.

Wang, Madeleine (2007) 'Informing patients: a "must" not a "maybe"', *Bulletin of the Royal College of Anaesthetists*, no 44, pp 2233–5.

Weale, Albert (1988) 'Principles', in Albert Weale (ed) *Cost and choice in health care: The ethical dimension*, London: King Edward's Hospital Fund for London, pp 19–24.

Webber, Matthew (2009) 'A patient's journey, electroconvulsive therapy', *BMJ*, vol 338, pp 169–70.

Weed, Lawrence L. (1997) 'New connections between medical knowledge and patient care', *BMJ*, vol 315, pp 231–5.

Whelan, Emma (2007) '"No one agrees except for those of us who have it": endometriosis patients as an epistemological community', *Sociology of Health & Illness*, vol 29, no 7, pp 957–82.

Whitcroft, Isla (2007) 'The cure that can kill', *Daily Mail*, 10 July, p 37.

Whitworth, Damian (2008) 'Can Lord Ara Darzi reform the NHS?' *Times2*, 1 April, pp 4–5.

Wilkie, Patricia (1998) 'RCGP patient liaison group: past, present and future', *British Journal of General Practice*, vol 48, no 434, pp 1623.

Wilkie, Patricia (2003) 'Experiencing care of the elderly in the community: a learning curve for carers', *Quality in Primary Care*, vol 11, pp 317–19.

Wilkie, Patricia (2008) 'Sixty years of the NHS: general practice and the patient 1948–2008', *Quality in Primary Care*, vol 16, pp 379–81.

Williams, Gareth and Popay, Jennie (2006) 'Lay knowledge and the privilege of experience', in David Kelleher, Jonathan Gabe and Gareth Williams (eds) *Challenging medicine* (2nd edn), London: Routledge, pp 122–45.

Williams, Helen (2003) 'Registrar's Report', *Bulletin of The Royal College of Pathologists*, vol 124, pp 33–4.

Williamson, Charlotte (1983) 'A study of the lay contribution to standards of non-clinical care in the National Health Service', DPhil thesis, University of York.

Williamson, Charlotte (1985) *Hearing patients' appeals against continued compulsory detention*, Birmingham: National Association of Health Authorities.

Williamson, Charlotte (1987) *Reviewing the quality of care in the NHS*, Birmingham: National Association of Health Authorities.

Williamson, Charlotte (1988) 'Dominant, challenging and repressed interests in the NHS', *Health Services Management*, vol 84, December, pp 170–4.

Williamson, Charlotte (1992) *Whose standards? Consumer and professional standards in health care*, Buckingham: Open University Press.

Williamson, Charlotte (1993) 'A model ahead of its time', *BMJ*, vol 307, p 742.

Williamson, Charlotte (1994) 'The eyes have it', *Health Service Journal*, vol 104, no 5385, pp 22–4.

Williamson, Charlotte (1995) Letter, 'Ensuring that guidelines are effective, give them to the patient', *BMJ*, vol 311, p 1023.

Williamson, Charlotte (1998) 'The rise of doctor–patient working groups', *BMJ*, vol 317, pp 1374–7.

Williamson, Charlotte (1999a) 'Reflections on health-care consumerism: insights from feminism', *Health Expectations*, vol 2, no 3, pp 150–8.

Williamson, Charlotte (1999b) 'Critical incidents and candour', *Royal College of Anaesthetists Newsletter*, vol 46, pp 113–14.

Williamson, Charlotte (2000a) 'Consumer and professional standards: working towards consensus', *Quality in Health Care*, vol 9, pp 190–4.

Williamson, Charlotte (2000b) 'A lay perspective on revalidation and the review of departments of anaesthesia', *Royal College of Anaesthetists Newsletter*, vol 51, pp 325–6.

Williamson, Charlotte (2001) 'What does involving consumers in research mean?' *QJM, Monthly Journal of the Association of Physicians*, vol 94, pp 661–4.

Williamson, Charlotte (2003) 'The patient perspective on information', in J. Alastair Lack, Anna-Maria Rollin, Gavin Thoms, Lucy White and Charlotte Williamson (eds) *Raising the standard: Information for patients*, London: Royal College of Anaesthetists and Association of Anaesthetists of Great Britain and Ireland, 2003, pp 73–6.

Williamson, Charlotte (2005) 'Withholding policies from patients restricts their autonomy', *BMJ*, vol 331, pp 1078–80.

Williamson, Charlotte (2007a) 'Radical patient groups', *AIMS Journal*, vol 19, no 2, pp 5–8.

Williamson, Charlotte (2007b) 'Lab tests: levelling down or up?', *The Bulletin of the Royal College of Pathologists*, vol 138, pp 63.

Williamson, Charlotte (2007c) 'How do we find the right patients to consult?' *Quality in Primary Care*, vol 15, pp 195–9.

Williamson, Charlotte (2008a) 'The patient movement as an emancipation movement', *Health Expectations*, vol 11, no 2, pp 102–12.

Williamson, Charlotte (2008b) 'Alford's theoretical political framework and its application to interests in health care now', *British Journal of General Practice*, vol 58, no 552, pp 512–16.

Williamson, Charlotte (2008c) 'The early days of the PLG', *Bulletin of the Royal College of Anaesthetists*, vol 50, pp 2549–50.

Willington, Sally (2007) 'Listen with mother', *AIMS Journal*, vol 19, no 2, pp 3–4.

Wilson, Edward O. (1975) *Sociobiology: The new synthesis*, Cambridge, MA: The Belknap Press of Harvard University Press.

Wilson, Judy (2005) 'Foreword', in Rob Baggott, Judith Allsop and Kathryn Jones (eds) *Speaking for patients and carers: Health consumer groups and the policy process*, Basingstoke: Palgrave Macmillan, pp ix–xii.

Winkler, Fidelma and Rosenthal, Helen (1988) 'Sexist practices in medical education – vaginal examination on women without consent', *Needle*, June, pp 10–11.

Winnicott, D[onald] W. (1964) *The child, the family, and the outside world*, Harmondsworth: Penguin Books.

Winyard, Graham (2003) 'Doctors, managers and politicians', *Clinical Medicine*, vol 3, no 5, pp 465–9.

Wollstonecraft, Mary (1975) *A vindication of the rights of women*, London: Penguin Books Ltd. (first published in 1792).

Wood, Bruce (2000) *Patient power? The politics of patients' associations in Britain and America*, Buckingham: Open University Press.

Woodward, Joan (2008) 'Enabling change', in Marci Green (ed) *Risking human security: Attachment and public life*, London: Karnac Books Ltd., pp 151–70.

Woolf, Steven H., Grol, Richard, Hutchinson, Allen, Eccles, Martin and Grimshaw, Jeremy (1999) 'Potential benefits, limitations, and harms of clinical guidelines', *BMJ*, vol 318, pp 527–30.

Wootton, David (2006) *Bad medicine: Doctors doing harm since Hippocrates*, Oxford: Oxford University Press.

Wright, Jane (2003/4) 'Things are changing', *AIMS Journal*, vol 15, no 4, pp 11–12.

Wrong, Dennis H. (1979) *Power, its forms, bases and uses*, Oxford: Basil Blackwell.

Yeo, Philip Y.K. (1990) 'Hysterectomy: a change of trend or a change of heart?' in Helen Roberts (ed) *Women's health counts*, London: Routledge, pp 113–46.

York Health Services NHS Trust (2001) *User involvement toolkit: Handbook for all staff working with patients*, York: York Health Services NHS Trust.

York Hospitals NHS Trust Infection Control Team (2004) *Pre-admission information regarding MRSA*, York: York Hospitals NHS Trust.

Young, Iris Marion (1990) *Justice and the politics of difference*, Princeton, NJ: Princeton University Press.

Young, Judith (1992) 'Changing attitudes towards families of hospitalized children from 1935 to 1975: a case study', *Journal of Advanced Nursing*, vol 17, no 2, pp 1422–9.

Zavestoski, Stephen, Brown, Phil, McCormick, Sabrina, Mayer, Brian, D'Ottavi, Maryhelen and Lucove, Jaime C. (2004) 'Patient activists and the struggle for diagnosis: Gulf War illnesses and other medically unexplained physical symptoms in the U.S.', *Social Science & Medicine*, no 58, pp 161–75.

Zimmerman, Mary K. and Hill, Shirley A. (2000) 'Reforming gendered health care: an assessment of change', *International Journal of Health Services*, vol 30, no 4, pp 771–95.

Zola, Irving Kenneth (1991) 'Bringing our bodies and ourselves back in: reflections on a past, present, and future "Medical Sociology"', *Journal of Health & Social Behavior*, vol 32, pp 1–16.

Index

challenges to 78–9, 83
coercion 27–9, 31, 61, 96
and 'real' patients 167–8
repressed interest holders,
    perception of 110, 122, 212, 213
standards, origins of 182–3
dominant interests 18–20, 22, 71
domination 14–15, 26–7

E

EACH (European Association for
    Children in Hospital) 50
Edwards, Nadine 76, 111
Elton, Charles x
emancipation 1, 2
emancipation hypothesis 40–1
emancipation movement, patient
    movement as 40–3, 205
emancipation movements 2, 4, 13–16,
    40, 214
empowerment 176, 179
Epstein, Steven 84, 88
equality 203–5, 209–10
    of moral agency 212–13
    of voice 204–5, 210
equity 94, 105, 111–12, 172, 200
European Association for Children in
    Hospital, *see* EACH
examining patients without consent
    30–1
experiential knowledge 70–1, 76–7

F

Freidson, Eliot 35
Freud, Anna 80
Fried, Charles 109, 113, 122
'The functioning of social systems
    as a defence against anxiety'
    (Menzies) 82

G

General Medical Council (GMC) 18,
    56, 57, 77, 118, 119, 133
general practitioners 19, 21, 171–2
    see also doctors
Gilbert, Hilary 133
Glaser, Barney G. 91
Goffman, Erving 34
Good Practice Campaign 171
Goodare, Heather 51–2
Goss, Roger 164
guidelines, withholding of 31–2

*Guidelines for referral of patients with
    breast problems* (Austoker) 119
gynaecology 43–4

H

haemophilia patients and HIV 72
Hancock, Sheila 63
Hardon, Anita 113
harm
    perceived 58–9
    risks of 118–19
Hartley, Elisabeth 83, 164
Haug, Marie R. 41
Health and Social Care Act (2001)
    188
*Health care politics: Ideological and
    interest group barriers to reform*
    (Alford) 16
health education 144, 152–3
health professionals
    patient representation,
        misunderstanding of 129
    and principles 187–8
    radical patient activists, influence of
        192–3
    and 'real' patients 166–8
    resistance to change 103–4
    secrecy 201–3
    see also clinicians; doctors; dominant
        interest holders
health service governance bodies, lay
    people in 136–8
healthcare, quality of 34–5, 209–14
Healthcare Commission 72, 189
Heilbrun, Carolyn G. 13, 33, 125, 204
Hill, Nancy 207
Hirst, Jenny 54, 55, 61
Hogg, Christine 91
home birth 118
Hospital facilities for children
    (HM(71)72) 83
Hospital for Sick Children, Toronto
    21
hospital visiting times 128–9
    children's wards 40, 50, 83, 102–3,
        111
    see also NAWCH (National
        Association for the Welfare of
        Children in Hospital)
Human Relations 82
humane care 189
Huntingford, Peter 164

N

National Association for the Welfare of Children in Hospital *see* NAWCH

National Childbirth Trust (NCT) 100, 163

National Confidential Enquiry into Patient Outcome and Death (NCEPOD) 202

National Consumer Council 133

NAWCH (National Association for the Welfare of Children in Hospital) 40, 49–50, 59, 102–3, 111

new knowledge, use of 80–4

new knowledge 70–4, 94

sources of 74–80

experiential knowledge 76–7

lay knowledge 75–6

lifeworld knowledge 76

medical knowledge 77–9

social movements 80

social sciences 79

use of

NAWCH 80–4

RAGE 84–9

NHS Plan (Department of Health) 188

Nietzsche, Friedrich 122

non-activist patients 130, 131, 206–8

non-radical patient groups 36, 37, 38–40, 148, 149

Northallerton Maternity Hospital 29–30

'Not listening to patients – is it instinctive?' (Hirst) 61

O

Obama, President Barack 3

The Observer 48, 49

obstetrics 43–4

'oppositional consciousness' 65

oppressed social groups 44–5, 129

oppression 14–15, 16, 29–30, 43, 45, 60, 61

The organisation of the in-patient's day (DHSS and Welsh Office) 93

organ-retention 'scandal' 15–16, 31

see also Alder Hey Hospital 'scandal'; Bristol Royal Infirmary 'scandal'

The origins of love and hate (Suttie) 82

out-patient clinics 212–13

overt coercion 29–30, 60–1

Oxfordshire Primary Care Trust 198

P

Pankhurst, Christabel 164

Parsons, Talcott 5

participation 186–7

patient activists *see* conservative patient activists; conservative patient groups; radical patient activists; radical patient groups

patient advocates 23, 132, 166

patient autonomy 5, 19, 60, 95–7, 107

and coercion 30, 31, 32

and core principles 97–8

and corporate rationalism 22

and information 88, 116

and medical ethics 98–100

and referral management 210–11

respect for 200

see also autonomy

patient-centred care 189–90, 195

patient groups 3–4, 24, 35–6, 42, 131–2

conflict and schism 135, 136–7, 148–9, 153–5

alignment with staff or with patients 142–3, 150–2

health education 140, 144, 152–3

representation 140, 141–2, 150

training for members 140, 145, 153

and conservative doctors 165–6

resources, lack of 24, 42

see also radical patient groups

patient information leaflets (PILs) 99, 115, 119

patient involvement 186–7

patient liaison groups (PLGs) 151–2, 169–71, 179–80

cultural issues 176–7

emotional issues 177–8

political issues 176

Royal College of Anaesthetists 173–5

Royal College of General Practitioners 169, 171–2, 200

Royal College of Pathologists 172–3

Royal College of Surgeons 169

patient movement 3, 7, 33–4, 204–5

birth of 34–5

conflict within 135, 136–7, 148–9, 153–5